THE AUTOIMMUNE ANTI-INFLAMMATORY DIET FOR BEGINNERS

THE AUTOIMMUNE ANTI-INFLAMMATORY DIET FOR BEGINNERS

DISCOVER THE DIET-DISEASE CONNECTION, LEARN BY SYMPTOM MANAGEMENT, AND EMPOWER YOUR HEALTH JOURNEY WITH THE TOP LIST OF ANTI-INFLAMMATORY FOODS AND HERBS.

T. SHERBROOK

TAS CREATIVE VENTURES LLC.

Copyright © 2025 by T. Sherbrook

Published by TAS Creative Ventures LLC

All rights reserved.

No part of this book may be reproduced in any form or by any electronic or mechanical means, including information storage and retrieval systems, without written permission from the author, except for the use of brief quotations in a book review.

Disclaimer

This book provides information on dietary management strategies for autoimmune conditions. It is intended for informational and educational purposes only and is not a substitute for professional medical advice, diagnosis, or treatment. Always seek the advice of your physician or qualified healthcare provider with any questions you may have regarding your health or medical conditions.

The dietary suggestions, lifestyle recommendations, and other information contained in this book are based on current research and traditional practices in managing autoimmune diseases. However, individual health needs vary, and certain recommendations may not be suitable for all readers. Before making any changes to your diet or healthcare routine, consult with a healthcare provider to ensure the information and suggestions are appropriate for your specific health needs and circumstances.

The author and publisher expressly disclaim responsibility for any adverse effects that may arise from the use or application of the information contained in this book. Reliance on any information provided in this book is solely at your own risk.

Created with Vellum

To my family and friends,
Thank you for being the pillars of love and laughter in my life and for filling my world with warmth and unwavering support. This book is a testament to the inspiration you've given me every day—thank you for lifting me up, cheering me on, and being the incredible people you are.

- To My Loving Family:
- My Husband, R. Sherbrook, is my rock at encouraging my journeys and helping me keep focused on my goal while still understanding the laundry isn't folded and doing it for me.
- My Son W. Sherbrook for understanding my distracted state of mind while still giving attention and snuggles.
- My Dad, W. Holt, for telling me years ago to make a book to help people like me.
- And to My Fabulous Friends:
- G. Kaiser for always filling the second mom role.
- H. Hopke, for being a huge role model and taking on the role of the sister I've never had with a pure heart.
- S. Orham for stepping in and being the missing sister I never had and godmother to our son.

- R. Worwood for filling a role as a sister and loving the weird me I am.
- M. Doyle for letting me be my weird self without judgment.
- Each of these strong women has been there for me through this whole book in one way or another. Whether looking at endless covers, the manuscript, or just listening to my exhaustion and lifting me up, they had my back.

With all my love and gratitude.

CONTENTS

Bonus Recipes & Extension of Chapter 5	xi
Introduction	xiii

CHAPTER 1   1
Understanding Autoimmune Diseases and Inflammation

The Science Behind Inflammation	5
Common Autoimmune Diseases and Their Symptoms	7
The Autoimmune and Inflammation Connection	11
The Role of the Immune System in Autoimmunity	14

CHAPTER 2   18
The Basics of The Autoimmune Anti-Inflammatory Diet

Foods to Avoid and Why?	21
The Importance of Whole Foods	24
Introduction to Healing Herbs	27
Creating Balanced Meals	29
Budget-Friendly Grocery Shopping	31

CHAPTER 3   34
Transitioning to the Autoimmune Anti-Inflammatory Diet

Preparing Your Kitchen for Success	34
Gradual Dietary Changes: A Phased Approach	38
Understanding and Handling Cravings	40
Deeper into Meal Prep and Batch Cooking Tips	42
Affordable Anti-Inflammatory Ingredients	45
Dining Out and Social Situations	48

CHAPTER 4 *Meal Plans and Recipes*	50
A Week of Anti-Inflammatory Breakfasts	50
Quick and Easy Lunch Ideas	54
Delicious Dinners for the Whole Family	56
Snacks and Smoothies for Inflammation	59
Comfort Foods Reinvented	61
Special Occasion Meals	64
CHAPTER 5 *Specialized Diets for Specific Autoimmune Diseases*	67
Managing Rheumatoid Arthritis with Diet	67
Dietary Strategies for Hashimoto's Thyroiditis	70
Eating Right for Lupus	72
Diet Tips for Multiple Sclerosis	74
Foods to Combat Celiac Disease	76
Nutritional Support for Psoriasis	78
Make a Difference with Your Review	83
CHAPTER 6 *The Holistic Approach to Managing Autoimmune Diseases*	85
The Role of Stress Management	85
Importance of Quality Sleep	88
Incorporating Gentle Exercise	91
Mindfulness and Meditation Practices	93
Natural Remedies and Supplements	96
Building a Support System	98
CHAPTER 7 *Empowering Your Health Journey*	102
Listening to Your Body	102
Keeping a Health and Food Diary	104
Real-Life Success Stories	107
Overcoming Initial Resistance	109
Staying Motivated and Consistent	111
Celebrating Small Wins	113

CHAPTER 8
Advanced Tips and Resources

Advanced Meal Planning Strategies	116
Sourcing Quality Ingredients	119
Exploring Anti-Inflammatory Spices and Herbs	121
Functional Foods and Their Benefits	124
Scientific Studies Supporting the Diet	126
Resources for Further Learning	128
Conclusion	133
Referances	137
Keeping the Journey Going	141

BONUS RECIPES & EXTENSION OF CHAPTER 5

https://docs.google.com/document/d/1LRxLxICD6-H0erU0aUmgT18xWuG_w9SSKAyhaZWqkEY/edit?usp=sharing

INTRODUCTION

∽

T. Sherbrook, I have always been an active, vibrant woman. Even not knowing all my life, I had had four autoimmune diseases all my life confirmed when I was thirty. I loved hiking, cooking for my family, and chasing after my child in the park. However, My life took an unexpected turn when I turned thirty. I began to feel constant fatigue, joint aches, and struggling to keep up with my activities. After numerous doctor's visits over the year, and it just progressively getting worse even with multiple tests repeatedly, I was finally diagnosed with four autoimmune diseases. The diagnosis was overwhelming, and I felt lost, unsure of how to manage my symptoms and regain my quality of life.

"Autoimmune Anti-Inflammatory Diet for Beginners" is a comprehensive guide designed to help you manage autoimmune diseases through diet and lifestyle changes. This book provides practical, budget-friendly advice that empowers you to take control of your health journey. By understanding the diet-disease connection and learning

INTRODUCTION

how to manage your symptoms, you can improve your overall well-being and regain your vitality.

Autoimmune diseases are more prevalent than many realize. According to recent statistics, approximately 50 million Americans suffer from at least one autoimmune condition. These diseases occur when the body's immune system mistakenly attacks its own tissues, leading to chronic inflammation and a range of debilitating symptoms. Conditions such as rheumatoid arthritis, lupus, multiple sclerosis, and Crohn's disease can significantly impact a person's quality of life, making it crucial to find effective ways to manage these conditions.

This book is organized into several vital chapters to guide your journey. The first chapter introduces the concept of the autoimmune anti-inflammatory diet, explaining its scientific basis and its benefits for symptom management and overall health. Subsequent chapters provide detailed information on specific autoimmune diseases, including foods to avoid and why, as well as beneficial foods and herbs tailored to each condition. You'll find practical tips for transitioning to this diet, budget-friendly meal plans, and resources for dining out while staying on track.

The autoimmune anti-inflammatory diet focuses on reducing inflammation in the body by eliminating foods that trigger immune responses and incorporating nutrient-dense, anti-inflammatory foods. Scientific research supports the effectiveness of this approach in managing autoimmune diseases. Following this diet can reduce symptoms, improve energy levels, and enhance your overall quality of life.

What sets this book apart is its emphasis on real-life testimonials and practical, actionable advice. Throughout

INTRODUCTION

the book, you'll find stories from individuals like Emily who have successfully managed their autoimmune conditions through diet and lifestyle changes. These testimonials offer hope and inspiration, showing you can regain control of your health.

My motivation for writing this book comes from my passion for helping beginners overcome the challenges of managing autoimmune diseases. With a holistic approach and an in-depth understanding of the diet-disease connection, I strive to deliver easy-to-follow guidance that anyone can implement into their daily routine. I want to empower you on your health journey, offering precise information on food sourcing and selection, symptom management tips, and practical advice for transitioning to a new lifestyle.

I understand the challenges you face, and I aim to reassure you that you are not alone. This book is designed to be approachable, empathetic, and informative, avoiding medical jargon or explaining it in simple terms. I encourage you to take control of your health journey using the tools and strategies in this book. Keep a food and symptom diary, join support groups, and seek ongoing education and support.

A holistic approach to managing autoimmune diseases is crucial. This means integrating dietary changes with lifestyle modifications and mental health strategies. By addressing all aspects of one's well-being, one can achieve better health outcomes and improve one's quality of life.

As you embark on this journey, keep an open mind and stay motivated. The path to better health can be challenging, but it is worth it. Take the first step by committing to read and implement the advice in this book. Together, we can work towards a healthier, inflammation-free life.

So, dear reader, let's begin this journey together. Let's

INTRODUCTION

explore the diet-disease connection, learn how to manage symptoms, and empower ourselves to achieve better health. The adventure awaits.

See Bonus link as well: https://docs.google.com/document/d/1LRxLxICD6-H0erU0aUmgT18xWuG_w9SSKAyhaZWqkEY/edit?usp=sharing

CHAPTER ONE

UNDERSTANDING AUTOIMMUNE DISEASES AND INFLAMMATION

When Sarah first noticed the persistent fatigue and aching joints, she brushed it off as the inevitable result of her busy lifestyle. She had a demanding job, two young children, and a home to manage. However, as the symptoms persisted and began to interfere with her daily life, Sarah decided to seek medical advice. After numerous appointments and tests, she received a diagnosis that changed her life: rheumatoid arthritis, an autoimmune disease. Sarah felt overwhelmed and confused, trying to grasp why her own body had turned against her. Many share her journey to understanding and managing her condition, and it's the cornerstone of what we'll explore in this chapter.

Autoimmune diseases are complex and often misunderstood. They occur when the immune system, designed to protect you from harmful invaders like bacteria and viruses, mistakenly attacks your body's cells. Think of your immune system as a high-tech security system in your home. Its job is to identify and eliminate threats, but in the case of autoimmunity, the system malfunctions and begins to target the very residents it is meant to protect. Typically, immune cells are adept at distinguishing between self and non-self, ensuring that only harmful invaders are attacked. However, this critical distinction breaks down in autoimmune diseases, leading to chronic inflammation and tissue damage.

Autoimmune diseases are more common than many realize, affecting millions worldwide. In the United States alone, over 50 million people suffer from one or more autoimmune conditions. These diseases can impact various organs and systems, making daily life a struggle. For instance, rheumatoid arthritis affects the joints, causing pain, swelling, and stiffness, while lupus can impact multiple organs, including the skin, kidneys, and heart. Hashimoto's thyroiditis targets the thyroid gland, leading to symptoms like fatigue, weight gain, and depression. The widespread nature of these diseases highlights the urgent need for effective management strategies.

There are over 100 autoimmune conditions, each with unique symptoms and challenges. Rheumatoid arthritis, one of the most well-known, causes inflammation in the joints, leading to chronic pain and mobility issues. Lupus, another common autoimmune disease, is characterized by a wide range of symptoms, including joint pain, skin rashes, and organ damage. Hashimoto's thyroiditis targets explicitly the thyroid gland, often resulting in hypothyroidism and its associated symptoms like fatigue, weight gain, and cold intolerance. These examples illustrate the diverse ways autoimmune diseases can manifest, affecting different parts of the body and requiring tailored approaches to management.

Despite their prevalence, many misconceptions surround autoimmune diseases. One common myth is that stress alone causes autoimmunity. While stress can exacerbate symptoms, it is not the root cause. Autoimmune diseases result from a complex interplay of genetic, environmental, and immunological factors. Another misconception is that alternative treatments without dietary changes can effectively manage these conditions. While some alternative therapies may relieve symptoms, a comprehensive approach that includes nutritional modifications is often necessary for long-term management. It's crucial to understand that no one-size-fits-all solution exists, and what works for one person may not work for another.

Understanding autoimmunity begins with recognizing the immune system's role and how it can go awry. In a healthy immune response, immune cells identify and attack pathogens, leaving healthy cells untouched. However, genetic predispositions, environmental triggers, and other factors can disrupt this balance, leading to the development of autoimmunity. For example, specific genes can make individuals more susceptible to autoimmune diseases, and infections or exposure to environmental toxins can trigger or worsen symptoms. By understanding these underlying mechanisms, we can better appreciate the importance of a holistic approach to managing autoimmunity.

The impact of autoimmune diseases on daily life cannot be overstated. Beyond the physical symptoms, these conditions can affect mental and emotional well-being. Chronic pain, fatigue, and other symptoms can lead to feelings of frustration, anxiety, and depression. Additionally, the unpredictable nature of autoimmune diseases, with their flare-ups and remissions, can make it challenging to plan and enjoy daily activities. Addressing these aspects of the disease can improve overall quality of life and well-being.

This chapter will delve deeper into understanding autoimmunity, its causes, and its impact on the body. We'll explore the different types of autoimmune diseases, their symptoms, and common misconceptions. By understanding these conditions comprehensively, you'll be better equipped to manage your symptoms and take control of your health. Whether you're newly diagnosed or have been living with an autoimmune disease for years, this chapter provides valuable insights and practical advice to navigate your health journey.

Autoimmune diseases are a medical curiosity and a significant public health issue. The increasing prevalence of these conditions underscores the need for greater awareness and understanding. You can make informed decisions about your health by educating yourself about the nature of autoimmunity and the factors that contribute to its development. This knowledge empowers you to take proactive steps in managing your condition, improving your quality of life, and reducing the impact of autoimmune diseases on your daily activities.

As we continue through this book, you'll find that managing autoimmune diseases involves more than just medications. A holistic approach that includes dietary changes, lifestyle modifications, and mental health strategies is crucial. By addressing all aspects of your well-being, you can achieve better health outcomes and improve your overall quality of life. This book is designed to guide you through this process, providing practical advice and support every step of the way.

So, let's begin by understanding what autoimmunity is, how it affects the body, and the common misconceptions that often surround these conditions. With this foundation, you'll be better prepared to navigate the complexities of autoimmune diseases and take control of your health.

∾

THE SCIENCE BEHIND INFLAMMATION

We often hear about inflammation, especially in health and wellness, but what does it mean? In simple terms, inflammation is the body's natural response to injury or infection. Imagine you get a cut on your finger. Almost immediately, the area around the cut becomes red, swollen, and warm. Acute inflammation is a short-term process that helps your body heal by sending immune cells to the injured area to fight off potential invaders. Acute inflammation is a protective mechanism, a rapid response to restore normal function.

However, not all inflammation is beneficial. Chronic inflammation is a different story. Unlike the short-lived, acute version, chronic inflammation persists over time, often causing more harm than good. The body sends inflammatory cells to fight without injury or infection. This prolonged inflammation can gradually damage healthy cells, tissues, and organs, leading to chronic diseases. You can think of chronic inflammation as a fire that continuously smolders, causing damage below the surface without being fully extinguished.

The triggers for inflammation are varied and can include infections, injuries, and autoimmune reactions. When your body encounters an infection, such as a virus or bacteria, it triggers an inflammatory response to eliminate the threat. Similarly, an injury like a sprained ankle will prompt inflammation to initiate the healing process. In the case of autoimmune reactions, however, the body mistakenly targets its tissues, leading to chronic inflammation. Additionally, environmental and lifestyle factors can play a significant role. Poor diet, lack of exercise, stress, and exposure to environmental toxins can all contribute to chronic inflammation.

The biological pathways that lead to inflammation involve a complex interplay of immune cells and signaling molecules. Cytokines are one of the key players in this process. These small proteins are released by immune cells and serve as messengers that regulate the intensity and duration of the inflammatory response. There are both pro-inflammatory cytokines, which promote inflammation, and anti-inflammatory cytokines, which work to reduce it. The balance between these opposing forces is crucial for maintaining health. When pro-inflammatory pathways dominate, chronic inflammation can ensue, leading to tissue damage and disease.

Chronic inflammation has far-reaching effects on health, impacting various systems in the body. It is closely linked to a range of common diseases, including heart disease, diabetes, and cancer. For example, chronic inflammation in the arteries can lead to atherosclerosis, characterized by the buildup of fatty deposits in the artery walls. This can result in heart attacks and strokes. Similarly, chronic inflammation is implicated in developing insulin resistance, a precursor to type 2 diabetes. Understanding and controlling inflammation can significantly improve overall well-being and reduce the risk of these chronic diseases.

Controlling inflammation involves addressing the underlying causes and adopting lifestyle changes that promote a balanced inflammatory response. Diet plays a critical role in this process. A diet rich in anti-inflammatory foods like fruits, vegetables, whole grains, and healthy fats can help reduce chronic inflammation. On the other hand, diets high in refined sugars, unhealthy fats, and processed foods can exacerbate it. Exercise is another powerful tool. Regular physical activity helps modulate the immune response and reduce inflammation. Also, managing stress through mindfulness, meditation, and adequate sleep can further support a healthy inflammatory balance.

Understanding the science behind inflammation provides a foundation for managing autoimmune diseases and improving overall health. By recognizing the difference between acute and chronic inflammation, identifying the triggers, and understanding the biological pathways involved, we can take proactive steps to control inflammation. This holistic approach helps manage symptoms and promotes long-term health and well-being. In the following chapters, we will explore practical strategies for implementing these principles into daily life, empowering you to take control of your health.

∼

COMMON AUTOIMMUNE DISEASES AND THEIR SYMPTOMS

Rheumatoid arthritis (RA) is a chronic inflammatory disorder primarily affecting the joints. Unlike the wear-and-tear damage to osteoarthritis, RA targets the lining of your joints, causing painful swelling that can eventually result in bone erosion and joint deformity. Common symptoms include tender, warm, swollen joints, morning stiffness that may last for hours, fatigue, fever, and weight loss.

RA typically affects the smaller joints, such as the fingers and toes. As the disease progresses, symptoms often spread to the wrists, knees, ankles, elbows, hips, and shoulders. The severity of symptoms can vary, with periods of increased disease activity, called flares, alternating with periods of relative remission. Common treatments include non-steroidal anti-inflammatory drugs (NSAIDs), corticosteroids, disease-modifying antirheumatic drugs (DMARDs), and biologics that target specific parts of the immune system.

Lupus, or systemic lupus erythematosus (SLE), is another autoimmune disease with a wide range of symptoms due to its ability to affect multiple organ systems. Its hallmark sign is a facial rash resembling a butterfly's wings unfolding across both cheeks. However, lupus can cause inflammation in the joints, skin, kidneys, blood cells, brain, heart, and lungs. Symptoms might include fatigue, fever, joint pain, stiffness and swelling, skin lesions that appear or worsen with sun exposure, fingers, and toes that turn white or blue when exposed to cold or during stressful periods (Raynaud's phenomenon), and shortness of breath. The diversity of symptoms and their intermittent nature often make lupus challenging to diagnose. Treatment strategies typically involve anti-inflammatory medications, immunosuppressants, antimalarial drugs, and corticosteroids to manage inflammation and immune system activity.

Hashimoto's thyroiditis is when your immune system attacks your thyroid, a small gland at the base of your neck below your Adam's apple. The thyroid gland is part of your endocrine system, which produces hormones that coordinate many of your body's functions. Hashimoto's disease is the most common cause of hypothyroidism (underactive thyroid). Symptoms often include fatigue and sluggishness, increased sensitivity to cold, constipation, pale and dry skin, a puffy face, hoarse voice, unexplained weight gain, muscle aches, tenderness and stiffness, joint pain and stiffness, excessive or prolonged menstrual bleeding, and depression. The primary treatment for Hashimoto's thyroiditis is hormone replacement therapy, which involves taking synthetic thyroid hormone to restore normal hormone levels and alleviate symptoms.

Identifying symptoms that may indicate an autoimmune disease is crucial for early diagnosis and treatment, which can significantly improve outcomes. Common symptoms include persistent fatigue, unexplained joint pain, skin rashes, and digestive issues. Fatigue in autoimmune diseases is often profound and not relieved by rest. Joint pain can be symmetrical, affecting both sides of the body, and may be accompanied by swelling and stiffness, particularly in the morning. Skin rashes, like the butterfly rash in lupus, can be a crucial indicator of an underlying autoimmune condition. Digestive issues such as abdominal pain, bloating, and diarrhea may signal conditions like Crohn's disease or celiac disease. Early diagnosis and treatment are vital to managing symptoms and preventing disease progression.

The diagnostic process for autoimmune diseases typically involves a combination of blood tests and imaging studies. Blood tests can detect markers of inflammation, autoantibodies, and other indicators of immune system activity. Standard blood tests include erythrocyte sedimentation rate (ESR), C-reactive protein (CRP), antinuclear antibodies (ANA), and rheumatoid factor (RF). Imaging studies such as X-rays, ultrasound, and MRI scans can help assess joint damage and inflammation. Specialists play a crucial role in diagnosing and managing autoimmune diseases. Rheumatologists specialize in diseases of the joints, muscles, and bones, while endocrinologists focus on hormone-related conditions. Dermatologists, gastroenterologists, and neurologists may also be involved, depending on the organs affected.

Consider the journey of Maria, who experienced severe joint pain and fatigue for years before receiving a diagnosis. She recalls, "I felt like I was constantly battling an invisible enemy. My joints ached, and I was always exhausted. It took multiple doctor visits, blood tests, and imaging studies before I was finally diagnosed with rheumatoid arthritis. Understanding my condition and finding the right treatment made a difference." Maria's story highlights the importance of persistence in seeking a diagnosis and the relief that comes with understanding and managing the disease.

Autoimmune diseases present many symptoms and experiences, making each individual's journey unique. Some may experience mild symptoms that come and go, while others face severe, debilitating conditions that significantly impact their daily lives. The diversity of symptoms underscores the importance of personalized treatment plans and a comprehensive approach to managing these complex diseases. By understanding the common symptoms and diagnostic processes, you can take proactive steps in seeking medical advice and managing your health effectively.

THE AUTOIMMUNE AND INFLAMMATION CONNECTION

Autoimmune diseases and inflammation are tightly bound in a complex relationship, where each can influence and exacerbate the other. Essentially, autoimmune diseases trigger an inflammatory response as the body's immune system mistakenly attacks its own tissues. This chronic inflammation, in turn, perpetuates and worsens the autoimmune condition. Imagine your immune system as a vigilant security team that has lost its sense of friend and foe. Instead of targeting only harmful invaders, it also attacks the body's own cells, leading to persistent inflammation. This flawed immune response is a hallmark of autoimmune diseases and explains why managing inflammation is crucial for symptom control.

Inflammation plays a significant role in the progression of autoimmune diseases. An inflammatory response is initiated once the immune system begins to attack the body's tissues. This inflammation is meant to protect the body, but in the case of autoimmunity, it becomes a chronic and harmful process. For instance, in rheumatoid arthritis, the immune system attacks the synovium, the lining of the membranes that surround the joints. This results in inflammation, causing the synovium to thicken and eventually leading to joint damage and deformity. Similarly, in lupus, the immune system can attack multiple organs, including the kidneys, heart, and skin, causing widespread inflammation and damage.

Autoimmune responses are the root cause of chronic inflammation in these diseases. When the immune system mistakenly identifies the body's own cells as foreign, it releases inflammatory cells and cytokines to attack these perceived threats. Cytokines are small proteins that act as messengers between cells, regulating the body's response to infection and inflammation. In autoimmune diseases, pro-inflammatory cytokines such as tumor necrosis factor-alpha (TNF-α) and interleukin-6 (IL-6) are overproduced, leading to chronic inflammation. This persistent inflammatory response damages tissues and organs, contributing to the progression of the disease.

Several specific autoimmune diseases clearly illustrate the connection between autoimmunity and inflammation. In multiple sclerosis (MS), the immune system attacks the myelin sheath that covers nerve fibers, causing inflammation and nerve damage. This inflammation disrupts the communication between the brain and the rest of the body, leading to symptoms such as muscle weakness, coordination problems, and vision issues. In Crohn's disease, an inflammatory bowel disease, the immune system targets the lining of the digestive tract, causing inflammation that can lead to severe abdominal pain, diarrhea, and malnutrition. These examples highlight how inflammation is both a symptom and a driving force in autoimmune diseases.

Understanding the inflammatory pathways involved in autoimmune diseases is crucial for developing effective treatments. One critical pathway is the NF-kB pathway, which regulates the immune response and inflammation. NF-kB is a protein complex that controls the transcription of DNA, cytokine production, and cell survival. When activated, it moves to the cell nucleus and turns on genes involved in inflammation. Another important pathway is the JAK-STAT pathway, which transmits signals from cytokines to the cell nucleus, influencing the expression of genes involved in immune function and inflammation. T-cells and B-cells, white blood cells, are also critical players in the inflammatory response. T-cells can directly attack infected or damaged cells, while B-cells produce antibodies that target specific antigens.

The long-term impact of chronic inflammation on autoimmune diseases is profound. Unmanaged inflammation can lead to the progression of the disease, causing continuous tissue damage and worsening symptoms. For example, in rheumatoid arthritis, ongoing inflammation can erode cartilage and bone, leading to joint deformities and loss of function. Chronic inflammation can also result in secondary complications. In lupus, prolonged inflammation can cause kidney damage, leading to lupus nephritis, a severe condition resulting in kidney failure if not adequately managed. Additionally, chronic inflammation increases the risk of developing other health issues, such as cardiovascular disease and osteoporosis.

Controlling inflammation is essential for managing autoimmune diseases and improving the quality of life. Reducing inflammation can slow disease progression, alleviate symptoms, and prevent complications. This can be achieved through a combination of medication, lifestyle changes, and dietary modifications. Anti-inflammatory medications, such as corticosteroids and biologics, are often prescribed to help manage inflammation. Adopting an anti-inflammatory diet rich in fruits, vegetables, whole grains, and healthy fats can further support the body's efforts to control inflammation.

Scientific evidence strongly supports the connection between autoimmunity and inflammation. Recent studies have shown that targeting specific inflammatory pathways can significantly improve outcomes for individuals with autoimmune diseases. For example, research on TNF inhibitors in rheumatoid arthritis has demonstrated their effectiveness in reducing inflammation and slowing disease progression. Expert opinions and consensus also emphasize managing inflammation in autoimmune diseases. For instance, the American College of Rheumatology recommends a comprehensive approach that includes both pharmacologic and non-pharmacologic strategies to control inflammation and improve patient outcomes.

Ongoing research continues to shed light on the mechanisms underlying autoimmunity and inflammation, paving the way for new and more effective treatments. Studies are exploring the role of the gut microbiome, genetic factors, and environmental triggers in the development and progression of autoimmune diseases. Understanding these complex interactions will help develop targeted therapies that can more effectively manage inflammation and improve the lives of those affected by autoimmune diseases.

∼

THE ROLE OF THE IMMUNE SYSTEM IN AUTOIMMUNITY

The immune system is an intricate network designed to protect the body from harmful invaders such as bacteria, viruses, and other pathogens. White blood cells, antibodies, and various immune organs like the thymus, spleen, and lymph nodes are at its core. White blood cells patrol the bloodstream and tissues, scanning for signs of infection or damage. Antibodies, produced by B-cells, are specialized proteins that recognize and neutralize foreign invaders. When a pathogen is detected, the immune system mounts a coordinated response to eliminate it, preventing infection and promoting healing.

In a typical immune response, when a pathogen enters the body, immune cells recognize it as foreign and mount an attack. For example, white blood cells identify the virus and release antibodies to neutralize it if you catch a cold. These antibodies attach to the virus, marking it for destruction by other immune cells. This process involves several steps: recognition, activation, response, and memory formation. After the pathogen is eliminated, some immune cells remain memory cells, providing long-term immunity against future infections by the same pathogen. This sophisticated system ensures the body can effectively defend itself against various threats.

However, in autoimmune diseases, this finely tuned system goes awry. Instead of targeting foreign invaders, the immune system attacks the body's cells, mistaking them for threats. Autoantibodies and self-reactive T-cells often drive this dysregulation. Autoantibodies are antibodies that mistakenly target the body's tissues, while self-reactive T-cells are immune cells that attack the body's cells. Several factors can trigger this autoimmune response, including genetic predisposition, infections, and environmental triggers. For instance, specific genetic markers are associated with an increased risk of autoimmune diseases, and infections can sometimes prompt the immune system to attack the body's cells mistakenly.

Diet and lifestyle play a significant role in modulating immune system activity. Vitamins D and C are crucial for maintaining a balanced immune response. Vitamin D, for example, helps regulate the immune system and reduce inflammation. It can be obtained from sunlight, foods like fatty fish, and supplements. Vitamin C, found in citrus fruits, bell peppers, and broccoli, supports the production and function of white blood cells. Probiotics, beneficial bacteria found in fermented foods like yogurt and sauerkraut, promote gut health, which is closely linked to immune function. A healthy gut microbiome can help regulate immune responses and reduce the risk of autoimmune flares.

Preventing autoimmune flares involves a combination of dietary and lifestyle strategies. Avoiding known triggers is critical. For many individuals, certain foods can exacerbate symptoms. Common culprits include gluten, dairy, and processed foods. Keeping a food diary can help identify which foods trigger symptoms, allowing you to avoid them. Stress management is equally important. Chronic stress can weaken the immune system and trigger flares. Techniques like mindfulness, meditation, and regular exercise can help manage stress. Regular medical check-ups and monitoring are also crucial. Working with a healthcare provider ensures you stay on top of your condition, adjusting treatments as needed and catching potential issues early.

Consider the case of John, who has been living with multiple sclerosis (MS) for several years. Through careful management of his diet and lifestyle, John has been able to reduce the frequency and severity of his flares. He noticed that certain foods, like dairy and processed meats, would trigger symptoms, so he eliminated them from his diet. John also incorporated more anti-inflammatory foods, such as leafy greens and fatty fish, into his meals. Additionally, he practices yoga and meditation regularly, which helps him manage stress. By making these changes and working closely with his healthcare team, John has gained better control over his condition, improving his quality of life.

The immune system's role in autoimmunity is both

complex and fascinating. Its primary function is to defend the body against harmful invaders, but when it becomes dysregulated, it can turn against the body, leading to chronic inflammation and tissue damage. By understanding the basics of the immune system and the factors that influence its activity, we can take proactive steps to modulate its response and prevent autoimmune flares. This holistic approach, which includes dietary changes, stress management, and regular medical care, is essential for managing autoimmune diseases effectively.

Knowledge is power in the journey to better health. Understanding the inner workings of the immune system and how it can go awry in autoimmune diseases equips you with the tools to take control of your health. Adopting a holistic approach that includes diet, lifestyle changes, and regular monitoring can manage your symptoms, reduce flares, and improve your overall well-being. This chapter has laid the foundation for understanding autoimmunity and inflammation, setting the stage for practical strategies to manage these conditions in the chapters to come..

∼

CHAPTER TWO

THE BASICS OF THE AUTOIMMUNE ANTI-INFLAMMATORY DIET

Imagine waking up one day and feeling like an entirely different person. Your energy is gone, your joints ache, and even simple tasks seem impossible. This was the reality for Mark, a once-active individual who found himself grappling with the relentless symptoms of an autoimmune disease. Mark's journey to regain his health began when he discovered the decisive role that diet could play in managing his symptoms. Through careful dietary choices, Mark started to see improvements in his energy levels, joint pain, and overall well-being. His story is a testament to the transformative potential of an anti-inflammatory diet.

Autoimmune diseases often present with common symptoms that can significantly impact your daily life. Joint pain and stiffness are frequent complaints, making it difficult to move freely and perform everyday activities. Fatigue and weakness can leave you feeling drained and unable to keep up with your routine. Digestive issues, such as bloating, abdominal pain, and irregular bowel movements, are also common, adding to the discomfort and disruption caused by autoimmune conditions. These symptoms can vary in intensity and duration, but they all share a common thread: inflammation.

One of the most effective ways to manage these symptoms is through dietary changes focusing on reducing inflammation. Incorporating anti-inflammatory foods like fatty fish, rich in omega-3 fatty acids, can relieve joint pain and stiffness. Salmon, mackerel, and sardines are excellent choices, as they contain high levels of EPA and DHA, which have been shown to reduce inflammation in the body. Additionally, adding turmeric to your meals can help alleviate joint pain. Turmeric contains curcumin, a compound with potent anti-inflammatory properties that can inhibit inflammatory pathways like COX-2.

Fatigue and weakness can be addressed by including energy-boosting foods in your diet. Leafy greens such as spinach and kale are packed with essential vitamins and minerals, including iron and magnesium, which support energy production and muscle function. Berries, particularly blueberries and strawberries, are rich in antioxidants that combat oxidative stress and improve overall vitality. Nuts like almonds and walnuts are also beneficial, providing healthy fats and protein to sustain energy levels throughout the day.

For digestive health, gut-healing foods are crucial. Fermented foods like yogurt, kefir, sauerkraut, and kimchi contain probiotics that support a healthy gut microbiome. These beneficial bacteria help reduce inflammation in the digestive tract and improve nutrient absorption. Fiber-rich foods such as whole grains, legumes, and fruits like apples and pears promote regular bowel movements and prevent constipation. Ginger is another powerful ally for digestive health, as it has been shown to reduce nausea and inflammation in the gut.

Let's explore some of the top anti-inflammatory foods that can be incorporated into your diet. As mentioned earlier, turmeric is renowned for its curcumin content, which has strong anti-inflammatory and antioxidant effects. Ginger, another potent anti-inflammatory food, contains compounds called gingerols and shogaols that reduce inflammation and pain. Leafy greens like spinach and kale are rich in vitamins A, C, and K, as well as folate and iron, all of which support overall health and reduce inflammation. Fatty fish, such as salmon, mackerel, and sardines, provide omega-3 fatty acids that have been extensively studied for their anti-inflammatory benefits.

The nutritional benefits of these foods extend beyond their anti-inflammatory properties. Turmeric and ginger, for example, are also known for their antioxidant activities, which protect cells from damage caused by free radicals. Leafy greens are nutrient powerhouses, offering many vitamins, minerals, and fiber that support cardiovascular health, bone strength, and immune function. Fatty fish are excellent sources of high-quality protein, essential for muscle repair and growth, and vitamin D plays a crucial role in bone health and immune regulation.

Understanding how these foods reduce inflammation can help you make informed dietary choices. The anti-inflammatory compounds in turmeric and ginger, such as curcumin and gingerols, inhibit inflammatory pathways and reduce the production of pro-inflammatory cytokines. Omega-3 fatty acids in fatty fish modulate the immune response by decreasing the production of inflammatory molecules like prostaglandins and leukotrienes. Leafy greens contain antioxidants like vitamin C and beta-carotene, neutralizing free radicals and reducing oxidative stress, a key driver of inflammation.

Incorporating these anti-inflammatory foods into your daily meals can be simple and enjoyable. Start your day with a refreshing turmeric tea made by simmering turmeric powder with a pinch of black pepper (which enhances curcumin absorption) and a splash of coconut milk. Prepare a vibrant ginger stir-fry with a mix of colorful vegetables and a serving of quinoa for lunch. Enjoy a delicious salmon fillet baked with a sprinkle of turmeric and a side of sautéed spinach in the evening. Simply substituting healthier oils like olive oil instead of vegetable oil can also significantly reduce inflammation.

By focusing on these anti-inflammatory foods and incorporating them into your meals, you can take proactive steps to manage your autoimmune symptoms and improve your overall health. The journey to better health begins with the choices you make each day. With the right **dietary strategies**, you can achieve a life with **less inflammation** and **more vitality**.

FOODS TO AVOID AND WHY?

Understanding which foods to avoid can be as important as knowing which to include in your diet. Certain foods are notorious for triggering inflammation, making your symptoms worse. Refined sugars, for example, are a significant culprit. Found in sugary snacks, sodas, and many processed foods, refined sugars spike your blood sugar levels, leading to an inflammatory response. This can exacerbate symptoms such as joint pain and fatigue. Trans fats, commonly found in fried foods and baked goods, are another proinflammatory food. They increase bad cholesterol (LDL) and lower good cholesterol (HDL), contributing to inflammation and putting you at risk for heart disease.

Processed meats, like bacon, sausages, and deli meats, are loaded with preservatives and unhealthy fats that can trigger inflammation. These meats often contain nitrites and nitrates, which have been linked to increased inflammation and a higher risk of chronic diseases. Additionally, they are high in advanced glycation end products (AGEs), compounds formed when meat is cooked at high temperatures. AGEs can promote oxidative stress and inflammation in the body, worsening autoimmune symptoms. Avoiding these meats can help lower inflammation levels and improve overall health.

Consuming pro-inflammatory foods doesn't just affect your symptoms; it has broader health impacts. A diet high in refined sugars and trans fats increases your risk of developing chronic diseases like diabetes and heart disease. These foods can also negatively impact your gut health by disrupting the balance of good and bad bacteria. A healthy gut is crucial for a well-functioning immune system, and an imbalance can lead to increased inflammation and a weakened immune response. Additionally, these foods can impair your body's ability to fight off infections, making you more susceptible to illnesses.

Common food additives and preservatives also contribute to inflammation. Artificial sweeteners like aspartame and saccharin, often found in diet sodas and sugar-free snacks, can trigger inflammatory responses in some people. Monosodium glutamate (MSG), a flavor enhancer used in many processed foods, has been linked to chronic inflammation and adverse effects on liver health. These additives can disrupt your body's natural processes, leading to increased inflammation and exacerbating autoimmune symptoms. Being mindful of these hidden ingredients can help you make better choices of food ingredients.

Reading food labels is crucial for avoiding hidden inflammatory ingredients. Look out for terms like "partially hydrogenated oils," which indicate the presence of trans fats. Ingredients like high-fructose corn syrup and artificial sweeteners should also raise red flags. When choosing packaged foods, opt for products with simple, recognizable ingredients. The fewer ingredients listed, the better. Whole foods like fruits, vegetables, and lean proteins are less likely to contain hidden additives that can harm health. By being vigilant about what's in your food, you can make choices that support your well-being.

To help you navigate the grocery store, here are some practical tips for choosing healthier packaged foods:

- Prioritize products labeled as **"organic"** or **"non-GMO,"** as they are less likely to contain harmful additives.

- Focus on whole foods and minimally processed options. For example, plain yogurt over flavored varieties, often containing added sugars and artificial ingredients.

- Compare labels and select products with lower sodium, sugar, and unhealthy fat content.

- You can make your own homemade versions of packaged foods, like homemade granola or salad dressings, to have full control over the ingredients.

Understanding the foods to avoid and why they trigger inflammation is vital in managing your autoimmune condition. By eliminating refined sugars, trans fats, and processed meats from your diet, you can reduce inflammation and improve your overall health. Awareness of common food additives and learning to read labels effectively will empower you to make better choices. These changes may seem challenging initially, but the benefits to your health and well-being are well worth the effort. This chapter will help you navigate these dietary adjustments, providing practical advice and tips to support your journey toward a healthier, inflammation-free life.

THE IMPORTANCE OF WHOLE FOODS

These foods are the cornerstone of an anti-inflammatory, as close to their natural state as possible, unprocessed or minimally processed, and free from artificial additives and preservatives. Fresh fruits and vegetables, for instance, are prime examples of whole foods. When you eat an apple or a bunch of spinach, you're consuming nutrients in their purest form, just as nature intended. Similarly, minimally processed grains and legumes, such as brown rice, quinoa, and lentils, retain their nutrient integrity, providing you with essential vitamins, minerals, and fiber.

The nutrient density of whole foods is one of their most significant advantages. Unlike processed foods, which are often stripped of their beneficial nutrients and loaded with empty calories, whole foods are packed with vitamins, minerals, and fiber. For example, oranges provide vitamin C, fiber, and antioxidants, all contributing to your overall health. In contrast, a glass of orange-flavored soda offers little more than sugar and artificial coloring. Whole foods lack artificial additives and preservatives, so you're less likely to consume substances that can trigger inflammation and other health issues.

Comparing whole foods with processed foods reveals stark differences. Processing often involves removing beneficial components like fiber while adding unhealthy ingredients such as refined sugars, unhealthy fats, and artificial chemicals. For instance, whole grain bread retains the bran and germ, providing fiber and essential nutrients. In contrast, white bread is made from refined flour stripped of these beneficial components. Processed foods like canned soups, frozen dinners, and sugary cereals are convenient but often come at the cost of added sugars, trans fats, and sodium, all of which can contribute to inflammation.

Incorporating more whole foods into your diet doesn't have to be complicated. Start by shopping for seasonal produce, often fresher and more affordable than out-of-season options. Visiting farmers' markets can be a great way to find high-quality, locally-grown fruits and vegetables. When shopping for grains and legumes, choose minimally processed options like whole oats, brown rice, and dried beans. These staples are versatile and can be used in various dishes, from hearty stews to refreshing salads. By focusing on whole foods, you can ensure that you're getting the most nutritional bang for your buck.

Meal prepping with whole foods can save time and help you stick to your anti-inflammatory diet. Consider making large batches of food-based salads and soups you can enjoy throughout the week. For example, a pot of vegetable soup made with fresh carrots, celery, tomatoes, and beans can serve as a nutritious lunch or dinner for several days. Similarly, preparing a large salad with mixed greens, quinoa, roasted vegetables, and a simple olive oil dressing can provide multiple healthy meals. Dedicating a few hours each week to meal prep can make it easier to eat well, even on your busiest days.

In addition to meal prepping, simple swaps can make a significant difference in your diet. Replace refined grains with whole grains, such as swapping white rice for brown rice or white pasta for whole wheat pasta. Choose entire fruits over fruit juices to avoid added sugars and retain the fiber content. Instead of snacking on processed chips or cookies, choose fresh fruit, nuts, or homemade snacks like roasted chickpeas. These small changes can add up, helping you reduce inflammation and improve your overall health.

Another practical tip for incorporating whole foods is to make your versions of common processed foods. For example, instead of buying store-bought granola, which often contains added sugars and unhealthy fats, you can create your own using oats, nuts, seeds, honey, or maple syrup. Homemade salad dressings are another easy swap; mix olive oil, vinegar, and your favorite herbs for a healthier alternative to bottled dressings. These homemade options allow you to control the ingredients and ensure you eat foods that support your health.

By focusing on whole foods in your diet, you can take control of your health and reduce inflammation naturally. Whole foods offer a wealth of nutrients that support your body's functions and help protect against chronic diseases. They provide the building blocks your body needs to repair and maintain itself, and they do so without the harmful additives found in many processed foods. Embracing a diet rich in whole foods can help you feel better, have more energy, and manage your autoimmune symptoms more effectively.

∽

INTRODUCTION TO HEALING HERBS

Herbs have been used for centuries to treat various ailments thanks to their potent anti-inflammatory properties. Consider basil, a common herb that you might already have in your kitchen. Basil contains eugenol, an anti-inflammatory compound that can help reduce swelling and pain. Beyond its culinary uses, basil also offers antioxidant benefits, protecting your cells from damage caused by free radicals. Thanks to its antimicrobial properties, it supports digestive health by promoting a balanced gut microbiome.

Oregano is another herb known for its anti-inflammatory effects. This powerful herb contains compounds like carvacrol and thymol, which have been shown to reduce inflammation and fight infections. Oregano is rich in antioxidants, which help protect your body from oxidative stress. It also supports digestive health by enhancing gut flora and reducing bloating and gas. Rosemary, with its distinct pine-like aroma, contains rosmarinic acid. This compound reduces inflammation by inhibiting the production of pro-inflammatory molecules. Rosemary also supports cognitive function and memory, making it a versatile addition to your diet.

Growing your herbs at home can be a rewarding and practical way to ensure you always have fresh, healing herbs on hand. You can cultivate various herbs with a spacious garden or a sunny windowsill. Choose pots with good drainage for indoor gardening and use a high-quality potting mix. Place your herbs in a sunny spot, as most herbs need at least six hours of sunlight daily. Water them regularly, but avoid overwatering, as this can lead to root rot. Plant your herbs in well-drained soil for outdoor gardening and space them appropriately to allow for growth. Basil, oregano, and rosemary are all relatively easy to grow, making them perfect for beginners.

When using these herbs in your cooking, the possibilities are endless. Basil can be used to make a flavorful herb-infused oil. Combine fresh basil leaves with olive oil and let it sit for a few days. They then drizzled infused oils over salads, grilled vegetables, or pasta dishes for an aromatic touch. Fresh herb salads are another fantastic way to incorporate more basil into your diet. Combine chopped basil with tomatoes, mozzarella, and a balsamic vinaigrette for a refreshing and anti-inflammatory dish. Oregano pairs wonderfully with Mediterranean dishes. Sprinkle it over roasted vegetables or mix it into a homemade marinara sauce.

Rosemary's robust flavor makes it a great addition to hearty dishes. Use it to season roasted meats or vegetables. You can also infuse olive oil with rosemary by gently heating it with a few sprigs and then letting it cool. This rosemary-infused oil can be used in salad dressings or as a dipping oil for bread. Try roasting potatoes with rosemary and garlic for a simple yet delicious side dish. The aromatic herbs will elevate the dish, and you'll benefit from their anti-inflammatory properties.

Incorporating these healing herbs into your daily meals enhances the flavor of your dishes and provides numerous health benefits. Growing your herbs ensures a fresh and readily available supply, allowing you to make the most of their potent anti-inflammatory and antioxidant properties.

Whether sprinkling basil on your salad, adding oregano to your pasta, or infusing oil with rosemary, these herbs can support your overall health and well-being.

∼

CREATING BALANCED MEALS

Creating balanced meals is vital to managing autoimmune symptoms and promoting overall health. A genuinely balanced meal includes protein, healthy fats, and complex carbohydrates. Protein is essential for muscle repair and immune function. Healthy fats, like those found in avocados and olive oil, support brain health and reduce inflammation. Complex carbohydrates, such as those in whole grains and vegetables, provide sustained energy and essential fiber. Fiber is crucial for digestive health, helping to regulate blood sugar and support a healthy gut. Micronutrients, including vitamins and minerals, play various roles in maintaining bodily functions and boosting immunity.

Portion control is also essential for balanced nutrition. It's easy to overeat, especially when dining out or snacking. Visual aids can help manage portion sizes. For example, a serving of protein should be about the size of your palm, while a serving of vegetables can be as large as your entire hand. Carbohydrates should fit into a cupped hand, and fats like cheese or nuts should be about the size of your thumb. These visual cues help you maintain balanced portions without measuring cups or scales. Overeating can also be avoided by eating slowly and paying attention to your hunger and fullness cues.

When composing anti-inflammatory and balanced

meals, variety and color are your best friends. Start your day with a breakfast like an avocado toast on whole-grain bread topped with a sprinkle of chia seeds and a side of berries. For lunch, consider a quinoa salad with colorful veggies like bell peppers, tomatoes, and spinach tossed with a lemon-tahini dressing. Dinner could be a piece of grilled salmon paired with roasted sweet potatoes and steamed broccoli. These meals look appealing and ensure you get a wide range of nutrients.

Practical meal planning can make sticking to an anti-inflammatory diet much more manageable. Begin by setting aside time each week to plan your meals. Create a shopping list based on your meal plan to ensure you have all the necessary ingredients. Batch cooking is another helpful strategy. Prepare large quantities of staples like quinoa, roasted vegetables, and grilled chicken, then store them in the fridge or freezer. This way, you can quickly assemble a balanced meal, even on busy days. Use glass containers to store your prepped food, as they keep the food fresh and make it easy to see what you have available.

Batch cooking can save you time and reduce the temptation to reach for unhealthy options. For example, cook a big pot of brown rice and portion it into containers for the week. Do the same with proteins like chicken or tofu and various roasted vegetables. Having these components ready allows you to mix and match to create different meals quickly. You can also prepare sauces and dressings in advance, like a homemade vinaigrette or a tahini-based sauce, to add flavor without extra effort. These small steps can make a big difference in maintaining a balanced, anti-inflammatory diet.

Finally, remember that a well-planned meal doesn't have to be complicated. Simple combinations of whole foods can provide all the nutrients you need. A bowl of mixed greens topped with chickpeas, cherry tomatoes, cucumber, and a drizzle of olive oil and lemon juice is both nutritious and delicious. Or try a bowl of oatmeal topped with fresh fruit, nuts, and a sprinkle of cinnamon for a warming, satisfying breakfast. By focusing on balance and variety, you can create meals as enjoyable as they are nourishing, supporting your health and well-being.

∼

BUDGET-FRIENDLY GROCERY SHOPPING

Eating a diet rich in anti-inflammatory foods doesn't have to break the bank. There are several strategies you can use to make healthy eating more affordable. One of the easiest ways to save money is by buying in bulk. Items like whole grains, beans, and lentils are often available in bulk bins at grocery stores, allowing you to purchase just the amount you need at a lower price per pound. Stocking up on these staples can save money and ensure you always have healthy options.

Choosing seasonal produce is another cost-effective strategy. Fruits and vegetables in season are often less expensive and taste better because they're at their peak of freshness. For example, strawberries in the summer or squash in the fall can be much more affordable than out-of-season options. Visit local farmers' markets or consider joining a community-supported agriculture (CSA) program to get fresh, seasonal produce at a lower cost. Not only will you save money, but you'll also support local farmers and enjoy various fruits and vegetables throughout the year.

Several affordable anti-inflammatory foods are easy to

find and incorporate into your meals. Beans and lentils are excellent sources of protein and fiber, and they're incredibly budget-friendly. You can buy them dried or canned, and the beans can be used in soups, stews, salads, and more. Frozen vegetables are another great option. They are often less expensive than fresh and can be just as nutritious because they are frozen at their peak ripeness. Stock up on frozen broccoli, spinach, and mixed vegetables to have on hand for quick and healthy meals. Choosing local produce over imported can also save you money. Locally grown fruits and vegetables don't have the added cost of transportation, making them more affordable. Plus, they are usually fresher and more flavorful.

Making smart substitutions can help you stick to your budget while eating anti-inflammatory foods. For instance, canned fish like sardines and salmon are often cheaper than fresh fish but still provide the same health benefits. Look for brands that pack fish in water or olive oil rather than soybean oil.

Planning your meals on a budget involves creativity and resourcefulness. Start by creating a weekly meal plan that includes affordable, anti-inflammatory foods. You might have oatmeal topped with frozen berries and a sprinkle of flaxseeds for breakfast. You could have lentil soup made with frozen spinach and canned tomatoes for lunch. You might have a stir-fry with frozen mixed vegetables, brown rice, and canned salmon for dinner. By planning your meals, you can make a shopping list focusing on budget-friendly ingredients, helping you avoid impulse buys and reduce food waste.

Utilizing leftovers creatively can also stretch your food budget further. For example, if you make a big pot of chili with beans and vegetables, you can enjoy it for dinner one night and then use the leftovers for lunch the next day. Add it to a baked sweet potato or serve it over a bed of greens for a different twist. You can add leftover roasted vegetables to many meals, like a frittata, for a quick and easy breakfast or lunch. Finding new ways to use leftovers can reduce waste and make the most of the food you buy. These strategies support your health and make healthy eating accessible and sustainable.

Eating well on a budget is about making informed choices that maximize nutrition and cost-effectiveness. The next chapter will explore transitioning to an autoimmune anti-inflammatory diet, offering practical tips and guidance to make the shift smooth and sustainable.

CHAPTER

THREE

TRANSITIONING TO THE AUTOIMMUNE
ANTI-INFLAMMATORY DIET

J*ane had always prided herself on her culinary skills, often experimenting with rich and flavorful dishes. But when she was diagnosed with an autoimmune disease, her doctor recommended an anti-inflammatory diet. Jane felt overwhelmed, unsure of where to start, and anxious about giving up her favorite foods. She understood that the kitchen contained items that could aggravate her condition. The transformation began with a simple yet crucial step: preparing her kitchen for success.*

∽

PREPARING YOUR KITCHEN FOR SUCCESS

The first step in transitioning to an anti-inflammatory diet is conducting a thorough kitchen clean-out. Cleaning the kitchen out involves removing foods that can trigger inflammation and exacerbate symptoms. Start by going through your pantry, refrigerator, and freezer. Look for items high in refined sugars, trans fats, and artificial additives. Common culprits include sugary snacks, sodas, processed meats, and packaged foods with long ingredient lists. Read labels carefully and discard anything that doesn't align with your new dietary goals. If you have unopened items, consider donating them to a local food bank. This way, you can help others while making room for healthier options.

Once you've cleared out the inflammatory foods, it's time to stock your kitchen with anti-inflammatory essentials. Begin with spices like turmeric and ginger, known for their potent anti-inflammatory properties. Turmeric contains curcumin, which reduces inflammation and pain. Ginger is another powerful spice that can help soothe your digestive system and reduce inflammation. Next, focus on pantry staples such as whole grains, legumes, and healthy oils. Brown rice, quinoa, and oats provide fiber and essential nutrients. Lentils and beans are excellent sources of plant-based protein. Opt for healthy oils like olive and avocado, rich in monounsaturated fats that support heart health.

Organizing your kitchen for convenience is another critical step. Arrange your spices and herbs in a way that makes them easy to access. Consider using a spice rack or drawer organizer to keep everything in order. Store fruits and vegetables in a way that maximizes their freshness. For example, keep apples and oranges in a fruit bowl on the counter. At the same time, leafy greens and berries are stored in the refrigerator for freshness. Use clear containers to store pre-cut vegetables, making grabbing a healthy snack or ingredient for your meals easy. This organization saves time and encourages you to regularly use fresh, wholesome ingredients.

Investing in the right kitchen tools and gadgets can

make meal preparation more efficient and enjoyable. High-quality knives and cutting boards are essential for chopping vegetables and prepping meat. Sharp knives make the task easier and safer, while sturdy cutting boards protect your countertops and knives. A food processor is a versatile tool that can save time and effort. Use it to chop vegetables, make hummus, or blend ingredients for soups and sauces. Similarly, a blender is invaluable for making smoothies, puréeing soups, and creating nut butter. These tools can streamline your cooking process and help you easily prepare nutritious meals.

Consider adding a slow cooker or Instant Pot to your kitchen arsenal. These appliances are perfect for batch cooking and preparing meals in advance. A slow cooker allows you to set and forget it, making it ideal for soups, stews, and chili. The Instant Pot, a multi-cooker, offers pressure-cooking, steaming, and slow-cooking functions. It's great for cooking grains and beans and even shredding chicken quickly. These gadgets can be game-changers in your kitchen, allowing you to prepare healthy, anti-inflammatory meals with minimal effort.

Silicone liners and storage containers are must-haves to enhance your meal prep experience further. Silicone liners are reusable, easy to clean, and eco-friendly. They are perfect for making egg cups, oat cups, and protein muffins. Storage containers help keep your meals fresh and organized, and glass containers are a great option as they don't absorb odors or stains. Steel containers are excellent for maintaining the temperature of your food, while mason jars are ideal for salads and smoothies. Reusable food bags are lightweight and convenient for packing snacks or storing leftovers.

With your kitchen well-prepared, you're setting yourself up for success on your anti-inflammatory diet. The clean-out process helps eliminate temptation and make room for healthier choices. Stocking up on anti-inflammatory essentials ensures you always have nutritious ingredients on hand. Organizing your kitchen for convenience makes meal prep more efficient, and investing in the right tools can transform your cooking experience. These steps support your dietary goals and make the transition smoother and more sustainable.

∽

CHECKLIST: Kitchen Clean-Out and Stocking Essentials

- Remove refined sugars, trans fats, and processed foods.
- Donate unopened items to a local food bank.
- Stock up on anti-inflammatory spices like turmeric and ginger.
- Fill your pantry with whole grains, legumes, and healthy oils like olive, coconut, and avocado.
- Organize spices and herbs for easy access, like turmeric, ginger, rosemary, oregano, and basil.
- Store fresh fruits and vegetables like blueberries, strawberries, apples, spinach, and kale for maximum freshness.
- Invest in high-quality knives, cutting boards, food processors, and blenders.
- Consider adding a slow cooker or Instant Pot.
- Use silicone liners and storage containers for meal prep.

By following this checklist, you can create a kitchen environment that supports your health and makes it easier to stick to your anti-inflammatory diet.

GRADUAL DIETARY CHANGES: A PHASED APPROACH

Transitioning to an anti-inflammatory diet can feel overwhelming, but a gradual approach can make it more manageable. By introducing changes step-by-step, you allow your body to adjust without feeling deprived or stressed. This method also increases the likelihood of long-term adherence. Rather than overhauling your entire diet overnight, focus on making small, sustainable changes that build upon each other. This phased approach reduces overwhelm and gives your body the time it needs to adapt to new foods and routines.

- **Start with Phase 1:** Elimination. This phase involves removing primary inflammatory foods from your diet, but tackling everything all at once is unnecessary. Begin by eliminating one category of inflammatory foods at a time. For example, you might start with refined sugars. These are found in sodas, candies, and many processed snacks. Cutting out refined sugars can have an immediate impact on reducing inflammation. Once you feel comfortable without these sugars, move on to the next category, processed foods. These often contain unhealthy fats, additives, and preservatives that can trigger inflammation. Focusing on one category at a time makes the process more manageable and less daunting.

- **Next comes Phase 2:** Addition of Anti-Inflammatory Foods. Once you've successfully removed primary inflammatory triggers, it's time to introduce foods that will help reduce inflammation. Start with easy-to-incorporate items like berries and leafy greens. Berries, such as blueberries and strawberries, are packed with antioxidants and fiber, making them a delicious and nutritious addition to smoothies, oatmeal, or salads. Leafy greens like spinach and kale are rich in vitamins and minerals that support overall health. You can add them to your meals, from green smoothies to sautéed side dishes. Try simple recipes incorporating these foods, such as a spinach and berry salad with a lemon vinaigrette, to make this phase easier.
- **Phase 3:** Maintenance and monitoring is about sustaining your new diet and observing how your body responds. Keeping a food diary can be incredibly helpful during this phase. Note down what you eat and how you feel afterward. Are your symptoms improving? Do you notice any adverse reactions to certain foods? Tracking your meals and symptoms allows you to make adjustments as needed. For instance, if certain foods still cause discomfort, consider eliminating them or reducing their intake. On the flip side, if you discover foods that make you feel terrific, make them a regular part of your diet.

Maintaining an anti-inflammatory diet requires ongoing effort and mindfulness, but it becomes easier with time. As you become more attuned to your body's responses, you'll better understand what works for you. This phase is about balancing and making dietary choices that support your health without feeling restricted. It's also important to stay flexible and open to adjustments. Your body's needs may change over time, and being willing to modify your diet accordingly can help you maintain long-term success.

Remember that it's okay to take it slow throughout this phased approach. There's no rush to make all these changes overnight. By transitioning gradually, you give yourself the best chance of sticking to the diet and reaping its benefits. Whether eliminating inflammatory foods, adding anti-inflammatory ones, or monitoring your progress, each step brings you closer to better health and well-being.

∽

UNDERSTANDING AND HANDLING CRAVINGS

Cravings can be one of the most challenging aspects of transitioning to an anti-inflammatory diet. They often have both emotional and physical triggers. Emotional triggers like stress, boredom, and emotional eating are common. It's not unusual to reach for comfort foods when anxious or down. Recognizing these emotional triggers is the first step in managing them. For instance, if you notice that you crave sweets when you're stressed, finding other ways to cope might be helpful, such as taking a walk, practicing deep breathing exercises, or engaging in a hobby that brings you joy. Emotional eating can become a coping mechanism, but by identifying your triggers, you can find healthier ways to manage your emotions.

Physical triggers also play a significant role in cravings. Nutrient deficiencies and blood sugar imbalances can lead to intense urges for specific foods. For example, a craving for chocolate might indicate a magnesium deficiency. At the same time, a desire for salty snacks could be a sign of a need for certain minerals. Blood sugar imbalances can cause sudden, intense hunger, leading you to reach for quick fixes like sugary snacks. Ensuring your meals are balanced with adequate protein, healthy fats, and complex carbohydrates can help stabilize your blood sugar levels and reduce cravings. Eating regular, well-rounded meals can prevent the extreme hunger that often leads to unhealthy food choices.

When cravings strike, having healthy, anti-inflammatory substitutes can make all the difference. For sweet cravings, reach for fruit instead of candy or baked goods. Fresh berries, apple slices with a sprinkle of cinnamon, or a small piece of dark chocolate can satisfy your sweet tooth without causing inflammation. Dark chocolate, with at least 70% cocoa, contains antioxidants and less sugar than milk chocolate. For savory cravings, consider nuts and seeds or roasted chickpeas. Almonds, walnuts, and pumpkin seeds provide a satisfying crunch and are rich in healthy fats and nutrients. Roasted chickpeas seasoned with your favorite spices make a delicious and crunchy snack that can curb cravings for chips or other salty treats.

Mindful eating practices can also help manage cravings. Slowing down and savoring each bite allows you to thoroughly enjoy your food and recognize your hunger. Pay attention to the flavors, textures, and aromas of your meals. This mindfulness can help you distinguish between physical hunger and emotional hunger. Before reaching for a snack, take a moment to check in with yourself. Are you eating because you're hungry or trying to fill an emotional void? By becoming more aware of your eating habits, you can make more intentional choices that support your health.

Practical tips for managing and reducing cravings include staying hydrated and drinking herbal teas. Sometimes, thirst can be mistaken for hunger. Drinking a glass of water or herbal tea can help determine if you're starving or just thirsty. Herbal teas, such as peppermint or chamomile, can also provide a calming effect, helping to reduce stress-related cravings. Ensuring that your meals are balanced with adequate protein and fiber can keep you full and satisfied, reducing the likelihood of cravings. Protein helps stabilize blood sugar levels, while fiber promotes satiety and aids in digestion.

Another effective strategy is to avoid restrictive diets that can lead to intense cravings. Allow yourself to enjoy your favorite foods in moderation. Completely cutting out certain foods can make them more appealing and increase the risk of binge eating. Instead, focus on incorporating healthy foods into your diet and practice moderation with less healthy options. This balanced approach can help you maintain a healthy relationship with food and reduce the likelihood of cravings.

DEEPER INTO MEAL PREP AND BATCH COOKING TIPS

Meal prep and batch cooking can be game changers for maintaining an anti-inflammatory diet, especially during busy weekdays. Preparing meals in advance saves time and reduces the temptation to grab unhealthy convenience foods. When you have ready-to-eat, nutritious meals waiting in the fridge, you're less likely to reach for that bag of chips or order takeout. Additionally, meal prep allows you to control the ingredients and portion sizes, ensuring that your meals align with your dietary goals.

Planning and scheduling your meal prep sessions is the first step. Start by creating a weekly meal plan. Decide what you will eat for the entire week's breakfast, lunch, dinner, and snacks. Write down the ingredients for each meal and create a shopping list. This list will help you stay focused at the grocery store and avoid impulse purchases. Allocate specific times for meal prep, such as Sunday afternoons or weekday evenings. Consistency in your meal prep routine will make it a habit, and soon, it will become a regular part of your week.

Batch cooking techniques can make meal prep more efficient. Cook large batches of grains and legumes in meals in multiple amounts. For example, prepare a big pot of quinoa or brown rice and portion it into containers for the week. These grains can be the base for grain bowls, stir-fries, or salads. Similarly, cook a large batch of lentils or beans. Use them in soups, stews, or as a protein source in salads and wraps. Preparing multiple servings of soups and stews is another excellent batch cooking strategy. A hearty vegetable and bean soup can be divided into portions and frozen for later use, providing a quick and nutritious meal.

Proper storage and reheating of prepped meals are crucial to maintaining their quality and nutritional value. Glass containers are ideal for storing prepped meals. They are durable, do not absorb odors, and can be used in the microwave or oven. Divide your meals into individual portions and store them in these containers. Containers make it easy to grab a meal in a hurry. When it's time to reheat, use safe methods to preserve nutrients. Avoid reheating food multiple times, as this can degrade its nutritional content. Instead, reheat only the portion you plan to eat. Microwaving is convenient and can change the nutrient value of the food, but if you prefer, use the stovetop or oven for gentler reheating.

Incorporating variety into your meal prep can keep things interesting. For instance, if you're preparing a large batch of roasted vegetables, season them differently for each meal. Use different spices and herbs to create diverse flavors. One day, you might have cumin and paprika roasted sweet potatoes; the next, you could enjoy garlic and rosemary carrots. This variety will prevent you from getting bored with your meals and help you stick to your anti-inflammatory diet.

Another tip for successful meal prep is to prep ingredients rather than complete meals. For example, chop various vegetables and store them in separate containers. Cook a few different proteins, such as grilled chicken, baked tofu, and boiled eggs. Mix and match these components to create various meals throughout the week. One day, you might make a salad with mixed greens, grilled chicken, and chopped veggies. You could use the same ingredients to make a wrap or stir-fry the next day. Prepping ingredients gives you flexibility and makes it easier to whip up a healthy meal.

Maximizing efficiency during meal prep sessions can save you even more time. Use kitchen gadgets like a food processor or Instant Pot to accelerate the process. A food processor can quickly chop vegetables or blend ingredients for soups and sauces. An Instant Pot can cook grains, beans, and even meats in a fraction of the time it takes on the stovetop. Utilizing these tools can make meal prep less daunting and more enjoyable.

Meal prep and batch cooking are potent tools for maintaining an anti-inflammatory diet. You can always have healthy, delicious options by planning and scheduling your sessions, using efficient cooking techniques, and properly storing your meals. This approach saves time and supports your commitment to a nutritious, inflammation-free lifestyle.

∽

AFFORDABLE ANTI-INFLAMMATORY INGREDIENTS

Transitioning to an anti-inflammatory diet doesn't have to strain your budget. Many affordable ingredients can provide the nutrients you need without costing a fortune. Beans, lentils, and other legumes are budget-friendly, incredibly versatile staples. They are rich in protein, fiber, and essential vitamins and minerals. You can use them in soups, stews, salads, or as a meat substitute in various dishes. Seasonal, locally grown vegetables are another excellent choice. These are often cheaper and fresher than out-of-season produce. Farmers' markets or community-supported agriculture (CSA) programs can be great places to find these affordable, nutrient-dense options.

Shopping on a budget requires a few innovative strategies. One effective method is buying in bulk, especially for grains and spices. Stores that offer bulk bins allow you to purchase just the amount you need, often at a lower price per pound. Stocking up on items like brown rice, quinoa, chia seeds, and spices like turmeric and cumin can save you money eventually.

Frozen fruits and vegetables are also cost-effective. They are typically less expensive than fresh and have a longer shelf life. Frozen berries, spinach, and broccoli are excellent choices that retain their nutritional value and can be used in various dishes.

Thoughtful meal planning can maximize the use of affordable ingredients. Start by planning meals around sales and seasonal produce. Check weekly flyers from your local grocery store and plan your meals accordingly. For example, if sweet potatoes are on sale, incorporate them into several weekly meals. Using leftovers creatively is another way to stretch your budget. Roasted chicken for dinner one night, then turned into chicken salad or added to a soup the next day. Multi-purposing leftovers saves money and reduces food waste, making your meal planning sustainable.

Homemade alternatives to expensive store-bought items can also help you save money. Making your salad dressings and sauces is a simple way to cut costs. For instance, a basic vinaigrette can be made with olive oil, vinegar, mustard, and herbs. Homemade alternatives save money and allow you to control the ingredients, avoiding added sugars and preservatives. DIY snacks like granola bars and trail mix are another great option. You can make a batch of granola bars using oats, nuts, seeds, and a natural sweetener like honey or maple syrup. Trail mix customized with your favorite nuts, dried fruits, and a sprinkle of dark chocolate chips for a satisfying and healthy snack.

Consider the versatility of beans and lentils as a cornerstone of your budget-friendly anti-inflammatory diet. A big pot of lentil soup can be a hearty meal for several days. Lentils can also be used in salads, mixed with vegetables and a light dressing for a nutritious and filling lunch. Beans, such as black beans or chickpeas, can be added to stews, made into hummus, or used as a base for veggie burgers. These legumes are affordable and packed with nutrients that support overall health.

Seasonal, locally grown vegetables can be the highlight of your meals. In the summer, tomatoes, cucumbers, and bell peppers make fresh salads or salsas. In the fall, vegetables like carrots, beets, and sweet potatoes can be roasted for a warm, comforting side dish. Shopping at farmers' markets or joining a CSA program can provide you with various fresh produce at a lower cost than grocery stores. Plus, you'll be supporting local farmers and getting produce that is often more flavorful and nutrient-dense.

Frozen fruits and vegetables are convenient and affordable for those who want to eat healthily without breaking the bank. Frozen berries can be added to smoothies or oatmeal, providing flavor and antioxidants. Add frozen spinach and kale to your diet by adding them to soups and stews or lightly sautéing them as a nutritious side dish. These frozen options are picked at peak ripeness and flash-frozen to retain their nutritional value, making them a great addition to your anti-inflammatory diet.

You can maintain a healthy, anti-inflammatory diet without overspending by incorporating these budget-friendly staples into your meal planning. Beans, lentils, seasonal vegetables, and frozen produce offer a wealth of nutrients and discount the cost of more expensive ingredients. Intelligent shopping strategies, creative use of leftovers, and homemade alternatives to store-bought items further help you stay within your budget. With some planning and creativity, you can enjoy a nutritious and satisfying anti-inflammatory diet supporting your health and well-being.

DINING OUT AND SOCIAL SITUATIONS

Eating out while maintaining an anti-inflammatory diet can be a challenge. Still, it's entirely doable with a bit of planning and mindfulness. When navigating restaurant menus, scan for healthy options like salads, grilled proteins, and vegetable-based dishes. Don't hesitate to ask for modifications to menu items. For example, request steamed vegetables instead of fries or ask for dressings and sauces on the side. Many restaurants are willing to accommodate dietary needs if you communicate them. Choose restaurants that offer various healthy options, such as those with Mediterranean or farm-to-table menus, which typically focus on fresh, whole foods.

Social gatherings can also pose challenges, but you can stay committed to your diet with some strategies. One practical approach is bringing a dish to share that fits your anti-inflammatory guidelines. Ensuring at least one healthy option is available allows you to introduce others to the benefits of your diet. Communicating your dietary needs to hosts in advance can also be helpful. Let them know about your dietary restrictions and offer to help prepare a meal that everyone can enjoy. Most hosts appreciate the heads-up and are usually willing to accommodate your needs.

Traveling doesn't mean you have to abandon your diet, either. Pack healthy snacks for the journey, such as nuts, seeds, and portable fruits like apples and oranges. These snacks can satisfy you and prevent the temptation to grab unhealthy options. When at airports or on the road, look for anti-inflammatory options. Many airports now offer healthier choices like salads, fruit cups, and grilled proteins. On the road, grocery stores can be a great resource. You can pick up fresh produce, whole grain crackers, and hummus for a quick and nutritious meal.

Dealing with peer pressure to stray from your diet can be tricky, but staying true to your dietary choices is essential. Practicing polite but firm responses to offers of non-compliant foods can help. You might say, "Thanks, but I'm following a specific diet for my health." Finding supportive friends or groups with similar dietary goals can also make a big difference. Surrounding yourself with people who understand and respect your choices can encourage you to stick with your diet.

Staying committed to your anti-inflammatory diet while dining out, attending social events, or traveling requires some planning but is entirely feasible. You can maintain your diet and support your health by making informed choices, communicating your needs, and preparing healthy snacks.

∼

CHAPTER
FOUR
MEAL PLANS AND RECIPES

When Lisa first heard about the anti-inflammatory diet, she felt hopeful and overwhelmed. She was excited about the potential benefits but unsure where to start. Breakfast, in particular, seemed challenging. Lisa had always relied on quick, sugary cereals or skipped the meal altogether. Anti-inflammatory breakfasts seemed daunting until she discovered simple, delicious options that were easy to prepare.

∾

A WEEK OF ANTI-INFLAMMATORY BREAKFASTS

Here's a seven-day breakfast plan with anti-inflammatory recipes to help you start your day with the right fuel. These meals are designed to be easy to prepare, delicious, and nutritious, supporting your health.

∾

- **Day 1: Overnight Oats with Chia Seeds and Berries**
  - Begin your week with a bowl of overnight oats. Combine rolled oats, chia seeds, almond milk, and a touch of honey in a jar. Stir well and let it sit in the fridge overnight. In the morning, top with fresh berries like blueberries and strawberries. The oats and chia seeds provide fiber, which helps with digestion. At the same time, the berries add a burst of antioxidants to reduce inflammation. To keep things interesting, rotate your fruit toppings. Try sliced bananas and a sprinkle of cinnamon one day and diced apples with a dash of nutmeg the next.
- **Day 2: Avocado Toast on Whole Grain Bread with a Side of Fruit**
  - Avocado toast is a quick and satisfying option. Mash a ripe avocado and spread it on a slice of whole-grain bread. Sprinkle with a pinch of salt, pepper, and a squeeze of lemon juice. For added flavor, top with sliced tomatoes or a poached egg. Serve with a side of fruit, such as an apple or a handful of grapes. The healthy fats in the avocado support brain health, while the whole grain bread provides sustained energy. Experiment with various hummus or nut butter spreads to engage your taste buds.
- **Day 3: Smoothie Bowl with Spinach, Banana, and Almond Butter**
  - Smoothie bowls are a fun and nutritious way to start your day. Blend spinach, a frozen banana, almond milk, and a spoonful of almond butter

until smooth. Pour into a bowl and top with granola, chia seeds, and fresh fruit like kiwi or berries. The spinach adds a dose of vitamins and minerals, while the almond butter provides protein and healthy fats. Pre-chopping fruits and vegetables can save you time in the morning. You can also prepare smoothie packs by portioning the ingredients into bags and storing them in the freezer.

- **Day 4: Scrambled Eggs with Turmeric and Spinach**
- Scrambled eggs are a classic breakfast; you can easily make them anti-inflammatory by adding turmeric and spinach. Whisk two eggs with a pinch of turmeric and cook in a non-stick pan. Add a handful of fresh spinach and cook until wilted. Serve with a slice of whole-grain toast. Turmeric contains curcumin, known for its anti-inflammatory properties, while spinach provides essential vitamins and minerals. For variety, try adding different vegetables like bell peppers or mushrooms.
- **Day 5: Greek Yogurt with Honey and Walnuts**
- Greek yogurt is a protein-rich breakfast option. Top a bowl of plain Greek yogurt with a drizzle of honey, a handful of walnuts, and a sprinkle of cinnamon. The yogurt provides probiotics for gut health, while the walnuts add healthy fats and antioxidants. You can also mix fresh or dried fruit for added flavor and nutrients. Preparing your yogurt toppings in advance can make your morning routine quicker and more enjoyable.

- **Day 6: Quinoa Breakfast Bowl with Blueberries and Almonds**
  - Quinoa isn't just for lunch or dinner; it makes a great breakfast, too. Cook a batch of quinoa and store it in the fridge. In the morning, warm a portion and top with fresh blueberries, sliced almonds, and a drizzle of almond milk. Quinoa is a complete protein, providing all nine essential amino acids, and is high in fiber. The blueberries and almonds add antioxidants and healthy fats. This meal is both satisfying and nutrient-dense.
- **Day 7: Sweet Potato Hash with Poached Eggs**
  - End your week with a hearty breakfast of sweet potato hash. Dice sweet potatoes and sauté them with onions, bell peppers, and a pinch of paprika until tender. Top with two poached eggs for a protein boost. Sweet potatoes are rich in beta-carotene, an antioxidant that supports immune health. The eggs provide high-quality protein to keep you full and energized. Preparing the sweet potato hash in advance and reheating it in the morning can save you time.

THESE BREAKFASTS TASTE great and provide a wealth of nutritional benefits. High in fiber, rich in antioxidants, and packed with healthy fats, they support overall health and help reduce inflammation. By preparing ingredients in advance and experimenting with different variations, you can keep your breakfasts exciting and enjoyable. With this plan, you'll start your day on the right foot and set the tone for a healthy, anti-inflammatory lifestyle.

REFLECTION SECTION: **Breakfast Journal**

Keep track of how you feel after each breakfast with a simple journal. Note down your energy levels, mood, and any changes in symptoms. Reflecting on these observations can help you identify which breakfasts work best for you and adjust as needed.

QUICK AND EASY LUNCH IDEAS

For those busy afternoons when you need a quick and nourishing meal, consider a quinoa salad with roasted vegetables and a lemon-tahini dressing. Start by cooking a batch of quinoa and roasting a medley of vegetables like bell peppers, zucchini, and cherry tomatoes. Toss the cooked quinoa and roasted veggies together, then drizzle with a dressing made from tahini, lemon juice, garlic, and olive oil. The quinoa provides a complete protein, the vegetables add fiber and vitamins, and the tahini dressing brings healthy fats and a burst of flavor. You prepare the salad ahead of time and store it in the fridge for a few days, making it an ideal option for meal prepping.

Another fantastic option is a chickpea and avocado wrap. Mash a ripe avocado and spread it on a whole-grain tortilla. Add a handful of chickpeas, some shredded carrots, and a few spinach leaves. Roll it up and pair it with mixed greens dressed in a simple vinaigrette. Chickpeas are an excellent plant-based protein and fiber source, while avocados add creamy texture and healthy fats. This wrap is quick to prepare and easy to take to work or school. Add some hummus or a sprinkle of feta cheese for a different twist.

Lentil soup with turmeric and ginger is a warm, comforting lunch that can be made in advance and portioned out for the week. Sauté onions, garlic, and ginger in a pot. Add dried lentils, diced tomatoes, vegetable broth, and a pinch of turmeric. Simmer until the lentils are tender, then season with salt and pepper. The lentils provide protein and fiber, while the ginger and turmeric offer anti-inflammatory benefits. This soup is perfect for a chilly day and can be easily reheated. For added variety, toss in some chopped kale or spinach towards the end of cooking.

For portable lunch options, mason jar salads are a convenient choice. Start with a base of cooked grains like quinoa or brown rice, then layer with colorful vegetables, such as cucumbers, bell peppers, and cherry tomatoes. Add a source of protein like grilled chicken or chickpeas and top with a simple dressing. When you're ready to eat, shake the jar to mix everything. These salads are not only visually appealing but also packed with nutrients. Another portable option is a bento box-style lunch, where you can include various anti-inflammatory snacks. Think sliced veggies with hummus, a handful of nuts, and fruit slices. These boxes are perfect for a balanced, on-the-go meal.

Batch cooking can simplify your lunch prep significantly. Consider cooking a large batch of quinoa or brown rice at the beginning of the week. These grains can serve as the base for various dishes, from salads to stir-fries. Additionally, roasting various vegetables can save you time and provide versatile ingredients for your lunches. Mix your favorite veggies with olive oil, salt, and pepper, then roast them in the oven. Store the roasted veggies in the fridge and use them throughout the week in salads, wraps, or as a side dish.

Including various ingredients in your lunches can keep things exciting and ensure you get multiple nutrients. For example, mix greens like spinach, kale, and arugula in your salads. Use a combination of fresh and roasted vegetables for different textures. Add some nuts or seeds for crunch and extra nutrition. With some planning and creativity, you can enjoy quick, easy, and delicious lunches that support your health and keep inflammation at bay.

∽

DELICIOUS DINNERS FOR THE WHOLE FAMILY

Imagine the satisfaction of serving a meal that nourishes your family and pleases their taste buds. Baked salmon with quinoa and steamed broccoli is a perfect example. Season the salmon with olive oil, lemon juice, salt, and pepper. Bake it in the oven until it flakes easily with a fork. Meanwhile, cook quinoa according to package instructions and steam broccoli until tender. This meal offers a balance of protein, healthy fats, and fiber. The omega-3 fatty acids in salmon are known for their anti-inflammatory properties. At the same time, quinoa provides a complete protein source, and broccoli adds a generous dose of vitamins and minerals.

Chicken stir-fry with mixed vegetables and brown rice is another family favorite. Slice chicken breast into thin strips and stir-fry in olive oil until cooked. Mix your favorite vegetables like bell peppers, broccoli, and snap peas. Stir in a simple soy sauce, garlic, and ginger sauce. Serve over a bed of brown rice. This dish is quick to prepare and can be customized to include vegetables. The combination of lean protein from the chicken and fiber-rich vegetables makes this meal satisfying and nutritious.

Try sweet potato and black bean tacos with cilantro-lime sauce for a fun and flavorful option. Roast diced sweet potatoes with a sprinkle of cumin and paprika until tender —warm black beans in a skillet with some garlic and onion. Fill whole grain or corn tortillas with sweet potatoes and black beans, then drizzle with a sauce from blended cilantro, lime juice, and Greek yogurt. These tacos are delicious and packed with fiber, vitamins, and antioxidants. The sweet potatoes provide beta-carotene, while black beans offer plant-based protein.

One-pot meals can simplify your dinner routine, making cooking and cleanup easier. A one-pot vegetable curry with chickpeas and coconut milk is a great option. Sauté onions, garlic, and ginger in a large pot, then add your favorite vegetables like carrots, bell peppers, and spinach. Stir in a can of chickpeas, a can of coconut milk, and curry powder. Simmer until the vegetables are tender and the flavors meld together. Serve over brown rice or quinoa. This curry is rich in fiber and healthy fats; the spices add a warming, anti-inflammatory kick.

Another one-pot wonder is slow-cooker beef stew with root vegetables. Combine chunks of beef with diced carrots, potatoes, parsnips, and onions in your slow cooker. Add beef broth, a splash of red wine, garlic, and thyme. Cook on low for 6-8 hours until the meat is tender and the flavors are well-developed. This hearty stew is perfect for busy days when you want a comforting meal waiting for you. The root vegetables provide essential vitamins and minerals, and the slow-cooking process enhances the flavors, making it a family favorite.

Kid-friendly options are crucial for ensuring everyone at the table enjoys their meal. Homemade chicken nuggets with sweet potato fries are sure to be a hit. Cut chicken breast into bite-sized pieces, dip in beaten egg, and coat with almond flour and spices. Bake until golden brown and crispy. Cut sweet potatoes into wedges for the fries, toss with olive oil and a bit of paprika, and bake until crispy. These homemade nuggets are a healthier alternative to store-bought versions, and the sweet potato fries add a nutritious twist.

Spaghetti with marinara sauce and hidden vegetables is another kid-approved dish. Make a simple marinara sauce by sautéing onions and garlic, then adding crushed tomatoes, Italian herbs, and a pinch of salt. Blend in cooked carrots and zucchini to sneak in extra veggies. Serve over whole grain or gluten-free pasta. The hidden vegetables add extra nutrients without altering the familiar flavor of the sauce, making it a win-win for both parents and kids.

Making family meals enjoyable and stress-free involves a few strategic tips. Encourage kids to help with meal preparation, whether washing vegetables, stirring a pot, or setting the table. Involving them in the process can make them more excited about eating. Creating a weekly meal plan with input from all family members ensures that everyone's preferences are considered. Weekly meal plans make meal times smoother but also help with grocery shopping and reducing food waste. The more engaged the whole family is, the more successful and enjoyable your meal times will be.

SNACKS AND SMOOTHIES FOR INFLAMMATION

Finding the right snacks can make all the difference when maintaining an anti-inflammatory diet. One easy and delicious option is roasted chickpeas with turmeric and cumin. Start by draining and rinsing a can of chickpeas, then pat them dry. Toss them with olive oil, turmeric, cumin, and a pinch of sea salt. Spread the chickpeas on a baking sheet and roast at 400°F for about 30 minutes, stirring occasionally until crispy. These chickpeas are crunchy and satisfying and packed with protein and fiber. Turmeric adds anti-inflammatory benefits, making this a perfect snack to keep on hand.

Apple slices with almond butter and cinnamon offer another simple yet nourishing snack. Slice a fresh apple and spread each piece with a thin layer of almond butter. Sprinkle a bit of cinnamon on top for added flavor and health benefits. The apple provides natural sweetness and fiber, while the almond butter offers healthy fats and protein. Cinnamon is known for its anti-inflammatory properties, making this combination both tasty and beneficial. This snack is quick to prepare and easy to take, whether heading to work or enjoying a day outdoors.

Carrot sticks with hummus are a classic snack that never disappoints. Peel and cut carrots into sticks and pair them with a generous scoop of hummus. You can make your hummus by blending chickpeas, tahini, lemon juice, garlic, and olive oil, or use a store-bought version if you're short on time. Carrots are rich in beta-carotene, an antioxidant that supports immune health, while hummus provides protein and healthy fats. This refreshing and filling snack makes it an excellent choice to curb midday hunger.

Regarding smoothies, nutrient-dense options can serve as both snacks and meal replacements. A green smoothie with spinach, avocado, and pineapple is a perfect example. Blend a handful of fresh spinach, half an avocado, a cup of frozen pineapple, and some coconut water until smooth. The spinach offers a wealth of vitamins and minerals, while the avocado adds creaminess and healthy fats. Pineapple contributes natural sweetness and a dose of vitamin C. This smoothie is refreshing, energizing, and easy to take with you on the go.

Berry smoothies are another fantastic option, combining the anti-inflammatory benefits of berries with other nutritious ingredients. Blend a cup of blueberries, a tablespoon of chia seeds, and a cup of coconut water for a delicious and hydrating drink. Blueberries are packed with antioxidants, which help combat inflammation, while chia seeds provide fiber and omega-3 fatty acids. Coconut water adds a touch of sweetness and hydration, making this smoothie a perfect pick-me-up any time of day. To keep things interesting, you can also experiment with different berries, like strawberries or raspberries.

For portable snacks, homemade trail mix is always a hit. Combine a mix of your favorite nuts, seeds, and dried fruit in a resealable bag or container. Almonds, walnuts, pumpkin seeds, and dried cranberries are all excellent choices. This trail mix is easy to carry and provides a balanced protein, healthy fats, and fiber mix. It's a beautiful option for a quick and satisfying snack on the go. Another portable option is energy balls made with dates, oats, and flaxseed. In a food processor, blend dates, rolled oats, flaxseed, and a bit of almond butter until the mixture sticks together. Roll into small balls and store in the fridge for a convenient and nutritious snack.

Balancing your snacks to maintain energy levels throughout the day is crucial. Combining protein, healthy fats, and fiber in each snack helps keep you full and satisfied. Avoid snacks high in refined sugars, which can cause energy spikes and crashes. Instead, focus on whole, nutrient-dense foods that provide sustained energy. For example, pairing apple slices with almond butter or enjoying a green smoothie with spinach and avocado ensures you get a mix of macronutrients that support steady energy levels and reduce inflammation. By choosing wisely, you can enjoy delicious snacks that align with your health goals and keep you feeling your best.

∽

COMFORT FOODS REINVENTED

Comfort foods often hold a special place in our hearts, but they can sometimes come with a heavy dose of inflammation. Fortunately, it's possible to enjoy these beloved dishes with healthier twists. Take cauliflower mac and cheese, for instance. Instead of using traditional pasta and heavy dairy, you can create a creamy, delicious dish with cauliflower and a cashew-based cheese sauce. Start by steaming cauliflower florets until tender. For the cheese sauce, blend soaked cashews with nutritional yeast, a touch of garlic, and unsweetened almond milk until smooth. Pour the sauce over the cauliflower and bake until bubbly. This dish provides the comforting creaminess you crave without the inflammation that dairy can cause. The cashews add healthy fats, while the cauliflower boosts your veggie intake.

Another comfort food favorite is sweet potato fries.

Baked sweet potato fries offer a nutritious alternative, unlike regular fries, which are often deep-fried and laden with unhealthy fats. Cut sweet potatoes into wedges, toss them with olive oil, paprika, and a pinch of sea salt, and bake them until crispy. Serve with a spicy aioli dip from Greek yogurt, lemon juice, and hot sauce. Sweet potatoes are rich in fiber, vitamins A and C, and antioxidants, making them healthier. The Greek yogurt in the aioli adds protein and probiotics, enhancing the nutritional value of this satisfying snack.

Chicken soup is a classic comfort food, especially when under the weather. An anti-inflammatory twist involves adding turmeric and ginger to the mix. Start by sautéing onions, garlic, and ginger in olive oil until fragrant. Add diced chicken, carrots, celery, and a generous pinch of turmeric. Pour in chicken broth and simmer until the vegetables are tender and the flavors meld together. Turmeric and ginger are both potent anti-inflammatory agents, making this soup not only comforting but also healing. The chicken provides lean protein, and the vegetables add essential vitamins and minerals.

Swapping out inflammatory ingredients for healthier alternatives can make a big difference in your comfort foods. For instance, whole grain or gluten-free pasta instead of white pasta can add fiber and nutrients to dishes like mac and cheese. Replacing heavy cream with coconut milk in soups and sauces reduces dairy and adds a creamy texture with healthy fats. Coconut milk is rich in medium-chain triglycerides (MCTs), which can support metabolism and provide a quick energy source. These simple swaps can transform your favorite comfort foods into nutritious meals that support your health.

Making comfort foods nutrient-dense involves adding extra vegetables and using nutrient-rich flour. For example, adding chopped spinach or kale to soups and stews can boost their vitamin and mineral content. These greens are rich in antioxidants and fiber, supporting overall health. Using almond or coconut flour in baking can add healthy fats and protein, making treats like muffins or pancakes more filling and nutritious. These flours are also lower in carbohydrates, which can help regulate blood sugar levels and reduce inflammation. By incorporating these nutrient-dense ingredients, you can enjoy comfort foods while nourishing your body.

Satisfying cravings for comfort foods without compromising health is enhancing flavors and using wholesome ingredients. Herbs and spices can elevate the taste of your dishes without adding extra calories or unhealthy fats. For instance, adding a sprinkle of fresh herbs like basil or cilantro to your meals can brighten the flavors and add a burst of nutrients. Healthy fats like avocado or olive oil can also satisfy your comfort foods. Avocado adds creaminess and healthy monounsaturated fats, while olive oil provides heart-healthy polyphenols. These ingredients enhance the taste and support your overall well-being.

Consider making a nutrient-dense version of your favorite dish when craving something rich and hearty. For example, try a whole-grain pizza crust topped with plenty of vegetables, lean protein, and a drizzle of olive oil. Or, make a comforting bowl of oatmeal with almonds, fresh berries, and a sprinkle of nuts. These dishes provide the flavors and textures you love while delivering essential nutrients. By focusing on quality ingredients and mindful preparation, you can satisfy your cravings and enjoy your comfort foods in a way that supports your health.

SPECIAL OCCASION MEALS

Celebratory meals can be delicious and anti-inflammatory, ensuring you and your guests enjoy the festivities without compromising health. One standout dish is herb-crusted lamb with roasted root vegetables. Begin by seasoning a lamb rack with fresh herbs like rosemary, thyme, and parsley, mixed with garlic and olive oil. Roast the lamb until it reaches your desired level of doneness. Meanwhile, prepare a medley of root vegetables such as carrots, parsnips, and sweet potatoes, tossing them in olive oil and seasoning with salt and pepper before roasting until tender. The lamb offers high-quality protein and omega-3 fatty acids, while the root vegetables provide fiber and essential vitamins.

For a vegan option, consider stuffed peppers with quinoa and black beans. Hollow out bell peppers and fill them with a mixture of cooked quinoa, black beans, diced tomatoes, corn, and spices like cumin and paprika. Bake the peppers until they are tender and the filling is heated. This dish is visually appealing and rich in plant-based protein and fiber. The quinoa and black beans offer a complete protein source, making this a satisfying and nutritious choice for your guests. The colorful presentation and robust flavors make it a perfect centerpiece for any special occasion.

Every celebration is complete with dessert, and a flourless chocolate cake with berry compote fits the bill perfectly. This decadent cake uses almond flour and dark chocolate to create a rich, moist texture. Serve it with a compote from mixed berries simmered with honey and a splash of lemon juice. The dark chocolate provides antioxidants, while the berries add a burst of color and additional health benefits. This gluten-free dessert satisfies your sweet tooth without causing inflammation, making it a guilt-free indulgence for special occasions.

It's essential to create a balanced and appealing menu when entertaining guests. Start with various appetizers, such as a vegetable platter with hummus or anti-inflammatory dips like guacamole and salsa. To accommodate different dietary preferences, offer a mix of protein sources, including meat and plant-based options. For the main course, include a range of side dishes that complement your main dish, such as a hearty salad with mixed greens, nuts, and a light vinaigrette. Various options ensure that all your guests can enjoy the meal, regardless of their dietary needs.

Holiday meals offer a unique opportunity to showcase anti-inflammatory dishes that are both festive and healthy. For Thanksgiving, consider serving a roasted turkey with a cranberry-orange relish. The turkey provides lean protein, while the relish, made with fresh cranberries, orange zest, and a touch of honey, adds a tangy, antioxidant-rich accompaniment. A butternut squash and sage risotto can be a comforting and elegant option for Christmas. Cook arborio rice with vegetable broth, adding roasted butternut squash and fresh sage. This dish is creamy and flavorful, with the squash providing vitamins A and C and the sage adding a fragrant touch.

Making special meals memorable involves using high-quality, fresh ingredients and incorporating seasonal and local produce. Fresh ingredients taste better and retain more nutrients. For example, using fresh herbs instead of dried ones can enhance your dishes' flavor and nutritional value. Seasonal produce, such as winter squash in the colder months or fresh berries in the summer, ensures that your meals are both flavorful and nutritious.

Creating a memorable special occasion meal doesn't have to mean sacrificing health for flavor. You can enjoy delicious and festive meals that support your well-being by choosing high-quality, fresh ingredients and focusing on anti-inflammatory options. Whether you're hosting a holiday feast or a celebratory dinner, these recipes and tips will help you create an unforgettable dining experience that everyone can enjoy. As you continue to explore the anti-inflammatory diet, you'll find that it's possible to celebrate life's special moments with nourishing and delightful meals.

This chapter has shown you how to create meals that bring joy and health together. Next, we'll explore the holistic approach to managing autoimmune diseases, integrating diet with lifestyle changes to support overall well-being.

CHAPTER
FIVE
SPECIALIZED DIETS FOR SPECIFIC
AUTOIMMUNE DISEASES

W*hen Megan was diagnosed with rheumatoid arthritis (RA), she felt a mix of relief and anxiety. Relief because she finally had a name for the pain and stiffness that had plagued her for years, and anxiety* because she didn't know how to manage it. Her doctor recommended a range of medications, but Megan wanted to explore natural ways to alleviate her symptoms. She began researching the role of diet in managing RA. She discovered that the foods she ate could significantly impact her inflammation levels and overall well-being.

∼

MANAGING RHEUMATOID ARTHRITIS WITH DIET

Finding the proper diet can make a difference if you have rheumatoid arthritis. One of the most effective ways to manage RA is by incorporating anti-inflammatory foods into your daily meals. Omega-3 fatty acids are particularly beneficial for reducing inflammation. Cold-water fish like salmon, tuna, and sardines are excellent sources of omega-3s. These healthy fats help control inflammation by reducing the production of inflammatory molecules in the body. Flaxseeds are another great addition; sprinkle them on your morning oatmeal or blend them into a smoothie for an anti-inflammatory boost.

Antioxidant-rich foods also play a crucial role in managing RA. Berries like blueberries and strawberries contain antioxidants that help neutralize free radicals, reducing oxidative stress and inflammation. These berries are not only delicious but also versatile. Add them to your breakfast cereal or yogurt, or enjoy them as a snack. Olive oil is another powerful anti-inflammatory food. It contains oleocanthal, a compound shown to reduce inflammation, similar to ibuprofen. Use olive oil in your salad dressings or drizzle it over roasted vegetables to reap benefits.

While incorporating anti-inflammatory foods is essential, avoiding foods that can exacerbate RA symptoms is equally important. Red meat is one such culprit. It contains arachidonic acid, a fatty acid that can promote inflammation. Processed foods high in refined sugars and trans fats are also best avoided. These foods can increase inflammation and contribute to weight gain, which puts additional stress on your joints. Instead, focus on whole, unprocessed foods that nourish your body and support your health.

In addition to making dietary changes, certain nutritional supplements can further support your RA management. Fish oil supplements are a convenient way to increase your intake of omega-3 fatty acids, especially if you don't eat fish regularly. These supplements have been shown to reduce joint pain and stiffness in people with RA. Vitamin D is another crucial supplement. It supports bone health and immune function, which is essential for managing RA. Many people with RA have low vitamin D levels, so it's worth discussing supplementation with your healthcare provider.

Meal planning can be challenging, especially when you're dealing with joint pain and fatigue. However, there are practical strategies to make it easier. Focus on easy-to-prepare meals that only require a little time or effort. For example, a simple stir-fry with vegetables, tofu, or chicken can be ready in minutes. Use a slow cooker to prepare stews and soups that can cook while you go about your day. Batch cooking is another helpful strategy. Prepare large quantities of anti-inflammatory dishes and freeze them in portions. This way, you'll always have a healthy meal ready, even when you don't feel like cooking.

Adding anti-inflammatory spices like turmeric and ginger to your meals can enhance their benefits. Turmeric contains curcumin, a compound with powerful anti-inflammatory effects. Add turmeric to your soups, stews, and smoothies for a golden health boost. Ginger is another versatile spice that can reduce inflammation and flavor your dishes. Use it in stir-fries and teas, or grate it over roasted vegetables. These spices enhance the flavor of your meals and provide additional support in managing RA symptoms.

By making thoughtful dietary choices and incorporating anti-inflammatory foods, you can take control of your RA symptoms and improve your quality of life. It's not about deprivation but about nourishing your body with foods that support your health. With some planning and creativity, you can enjoy delicious meals that help manage your condition.

DIETARY STRATEGIES FOR HASHIMOTO'S THYROIDITIS

Living with Hashimoto's thyroiditis can be challenging, but the proper diet can support thyroid function and improve overall health. One critical nutrient for thyroid health is selenium. Brazil nuts are an excellent source of selenium; just one or two nuts daily can meet your daily requirements. Eggs are another great option, providing both selenium and essential amino acids and vitamins. Including these foods in your diet can help support your thyroid and overall well-being.

Iodine is another crucial nutrient for thyroid function. Seaweed, such as nori, kelp, and wakame, is rich in iodine and easily added to soups, salads, or sushi rolls. If you're not a fan of seaweed, iodized salt is a convenient alternative. Using iodized salt in your cooking can help ensure you get enough iodine to support your thyroid. Zinc is also essential for thyroid health; foods like chickpeas and pumpkin seeds are excellent sources. We can add foods high in zinc to salads, soups, or enjoyed as snacks to help maintain adequate zinc levels.

While incorporating nutrient-rich foods is important, avoiding foods that can interfere with thyroid function is equally essential. Cruciferous vegetables, such as broccoli, kale, and Brussels sprouts, contain goitrogens, which can disrupt thyroid function when consumed in large amounts. It doesn't mean you have to eliminate them. Still, it's best to consume them in moderation and preferably cooked, which reduces their goitrogenic effect. Soy products are another group to be cautious with. They contain compounds that can interfere with thyroid hormone production, so limiting your intake of soy milk, tofu, and other soy-based products is wise.

Maintaining stable blood sugar levels is crucial for managing Hashimoto's thyroiditis. Fluctuations in blood sugar can stress the thyroid and exacerbate symptoms. Incorporating complex carbohydrates into your diet can help maintain steady blood sugar levels. Foods like whole grains, legumes, and starchy vegetables provide a slow and steady release of glucose into the bloodstream, preventing spikes and crashes. High-fiber foods such as oats, lentils, and beans are particularly beneficial as they promote satiety and help regulate blood sugar levels.

A balanced diet tailored to support thyroid health can make a significant difference in managing Hashimoto's thyroiditis. Here's a sample meal plan to help you start: Enjoy a bowl of Greek yogurt topped with chia seeds and fresh berries for breakfast. The yogurt provides protein and probiotics, while the chia seeds add fiber and omega-3 fatty acids. The berries are rich in antioxidants, supporting overall health. Lunch could be a quinoa salad with mixed greens, grilled chicken, and a light vinaigrette. Quinoa is a complete protein that contains essential amino acids, while the greens provide vitamins and minerals. The grilled chicken adds lean protein, making it a satisfying and nutritious meal.

Dinner might include baked cod with roasted sweet potatoes and steamed broccoli. Cod is a rich source of iodine and lean protein. Sweet potatoes provide complex carbohydrates and are high in vitamin A. Steaming the broccoli helps reduce its goitrogen content while retaining its nutritional benefits. This meal is balanced and supports thyroid health and overall well-being.

You can effectively manage Hashimoto's thyroiditis by

focusing on nutrient-rich foods, avoiding those that can interfere with thyroid function, and maintaining stable blood sugar levels. These dietary strategies and regular medical care can help you feel better and improve your quality of life.

EATING RIGHT FOR LUPUS

Navigating life with lupus can be challenging, but the right dietary choices can help manage symptoms and support overall health. Lupus is a chronic autoimmune disease affecting various body parts, causing inflammation, pain, and tissue damage. Adopting an anti-inflammatory diet is one of the most effective ways to manage lupus. Incorporating fatty fish like mackerel and sardines into your meals can be particularly beneficial. These fish are rich in omega-3 fatty acids, which help reduce inflammation and support heart health. Adding these to your weekly diet can make a noticeable difference in managing lupus symptoms.

Colorful vegetables and fruits are also crucial for those with lupus. These foods are packed with antioxidants, which help combat oxidative stress and reduce inflammation. Think of your plate as a canvas and aim to fill it with a rainbow of colors. Carrots, bell peppers, spinach, and berries are excellent choices. These vibrant foods provide essential vitamins and minerals that support immune function and overall well-being. Vibrant foods can easily be incorporated into salads, smoothies, or as side dishes to your main meals.

While adding anti-inflammatory foods is essential, avoiding foods that may trigger lupus flare-ups is equally crucial. Alfalfa sprouts are a food that can activate the immune system and exacerbate symptoms—limiting trigger foods like whole high-fat dairy products and butter. These foods are high in saturated fats, increasing inflammation and negatively impacting heart health. Opt for healthier fats like olive oil or avocado, which provide anti-inflammatory benefits without the drawbacks of saturated fats.

Supporting immune function is essential for managing lupus without exacerbating the condition. Vitamin E is a powerful antioxidant that can support immune health. Foods like almonds and sunflower seeds are rich in vitamin E and can be easily added to your diet. Sprinkle sunflower seeds on your salads, or enjoy a handful of almonds as a snack. Probiotic-rich foods like kefir and sauerkraut are also beneficial. They promote a healthy gut microbiome, which is crucial to immune function. A healthy gut can help regulate inflammation and improve overall health.

Staying hydrated is another crucial aspect of managing lupus. Drinking plenty of water helps flush out toxins and supports kidney function, which is often affected by lupus. Aim to drink half your body weight in ounces of water a day. Herbal teas can be a great addition to your hydration routine. Teas like chamomile, ginger, and peppermint have anti-inflammatory properties and can be soothing for the digestive system. Including detoxifying foods like cilantro and beets can further support your body's natural detoxification processes. Cilantro can be added to salads, salsas, or smoothies, while beets can be roasted, juiced, or added to salads.

To make these dietary changes more manageable, plan your meals in advance and keep your kitchen stocked with anti-inflammatory foods. Prepare large batches of soups and stews incorporating fatty fish, colorful vegetables, and detoxifying herbs. These can be stored in the fridge or freezer for easy access during busy days. Taking proactive steps to manage your diet can help control lupus symptoms and improve your quality of life.

It's also helpful to keep a food and symptom diary. Track what you eat and how you feel afterward. Tracking what you eat can help you identify foods that trigger symptoms and those that help alleviate them. Over time, you'll develop a personalized diet plan that best supports your health. Remember, managing lupus is a continuous process. Still, with the right dietary choices, you can take significant steps towards feeling better and living healthier. Keep experimenting with new recipes and find joy in nourishing your body with foods that support your well-being.

∽

DIET TIPS FOR MULTIPLE SCLEROSIS

When dealing with Multiple Sclerosis (MS), diet can play a crucial role in managing inflammation and supporting overall health. One of the best ways to reduce inflammation is by incorporating leafy greens such as spinach and kale into your meals. These greens are rich in antioxidants and vitamins that help combat oxidative stress. They are also high in fiber, which supports digestive health. Adding a handful of spinach to your morning smoothie or a serving of kale to your salads can significantly reduce inflammation.

Berries are another excellent choice for anyone managing MS. Blueberries, strawberries, and raspberries are packed with antioxidants, specifically flavonoids, that help neutralize free radicals. Free radicals can cause cellular damage and inflammation, so keeping them in check is vital. Enjoy fresh or frozen berries and added to various dishes, from breakfast bowls to desserts. Their natural sweetness also makes them a healthy alternative to sugary snacks, which can exacerbate MS symptoms.

It's equally important to avoid foods that can worsen MS symptoms. High-sodium foods are a significant concern. Too much sodium can increase blood pressure and contribute to fluid retention, negatively affecting your health. Processed foods, canned soups, and fast food are often high in sodium, so limiting these items is best. Instead, choose fresh, whole foods and season your meals with herbs and spices rather than salt. Refined sugars are another culprit. They can lead to spikes and crashes in blood sugar levels, contributing to fatigue, a common symptom in MS. Reducing your sugary snacks, sodas, and sweets can help maintain more stable energy levels.

Supporting brain health is crucial for managing MS, and certain nutrients can make a big difference. Omega-3 fatty acids are known for their anti-inflammatory properties and role in brain health. Fish oil supplements or chia seeds are excellent sources of omega-3s. Including these in your diet can help reduce inflammation and support cognitive function. Antioxidants from dark chocolate and green tea can also benefit brain health. Dark chocolate, in moderation, provides flavonoids that protect brain cells from oxidative stress. Green tea contains catechins, which have been shown to improve brain function and reduce the risk of neurodegenerative diseases.

Meal planning can help manage energy levels throughout the day. Instead of sticking to three large meals, consider eating smaller, more frequent meals. This approach can help maintain steady energy levels and prevent the fatigue that often accompanies MS. Including protein-rich snacks like nuts, seeds, and yogurt can keep you fueled between meals. For breakfast, you might have a smoothie with spinach, chia seeds, and berries. Mid-morning, a handful of almonds can provide a protein boost. Lunch could be a salad with leafy greens, grilled chicken, and a light vinaigrette. An afternoon snack of Greek yogurt with a drizzle of honey can keep you going until dinner, which might include steamed fish, quinoa, and roasted vegetables.

Incorporating these dietary strategies can make a significant difference in managing Multiple Sclerosis. By focusing on anti-inflammatory foods, avoiding those that can worsen symptoms, and supporting brain health with the proper nutrients, you can take proactive steps towards better health. Meal planning and small, frequent meals can help maintain energy levels, making it easier to manage the daily challenges of MS. Keep experimenting with different foods and recipes to find what works best for you and enjoy the benefits of a well-balanced, anti-inflammatory diet.

∽

FOODS TO COMBAT CELIAC DISEASE

Living with celiac disease means adhering to a strict gluten-free diet, which can feel daunting at first. However, understanding the basics can make the transition smoother. Gluten is a protein found in wheat, barley, rye, and their derivatives. It gives dough its elasticity and helps it rise. For those with celiac disease, consuming gluten triggers an immune response that damages the small intestine, leading to nutrient malabsorption and a host of symptoms. Ensuring your gluten-free diet is crucial to managing the condition and maintaining your health.

Naturally, gluten-free grains are a great starting point. Quinoa and rice are excellent staples in various dishes. Quinoa is gluten-free and packed with protein and fiber, making it a nutritious meal addition. Rice, mainly brown rice, provides essential vitamins and minerals and is a versatile base for many recipes. Gluten-free flours like almond and coconut flour are perfect for baking and cooking. These flours offer a different texture and flavor than wheat flour but are just as versatile. Almond flour adds a nutty flavor and is rich in protein and healthy fats, while coconut flour is high in fiber and has a subtle sweetness.

Hidden sources of gluten can sneak into your diet if you need to be more careful. Processed foods often contain additives like malt, modified food starch, and soy sauce, which can all contain gluten. It's essential to read labels meticulously. Some medications and supplements may also contain gluten as a filler, so always check with your pharmacist. Cross-contamination is another risk, especially in shared kitchens. Using separate utensils, toasters, and cutting boards for gluten-free foods can help reduce this risk. Keeping your gluten-free foods separate from gluten-containing items can also prevent accidental contamination.

To ensure balanced nutrition on a gluten-free diet, focus on nutrient-dense foods. Legumes, such as lentils and chickpeas, are excellent sources of protein and fiber. You can place gluten-free grains into soups, stews, and salads or even make them into dips like hummus. Leafy greens and colorful vegetables should be a significant part of your diet. These foods are rich in vitamins, minerals, and antioxidants that support overall health. Spinach, kale, bell peppers, and carrots are significant options that can be used in various recipes, from salads to stir-fries. Including various vegetables ensures you get a range of nutrients and keeps your meals interesting.

Here's a sample gluten-free meal plan to help you get started. Enjoy a smoothie made with spinach, banana, and almond milk for breakfast. This gluten-free smoothie is packed with vitamins and minerals to start your day. For lunch, a lentil soup with a side of mixed greens makes a hearty and nutritious meal. Lentils provide protein and fiber, while mixed greens add essential vitamins and minerals. For dinner, try grilled chicken with roasted vegetables and quinoa. The chicken offers lean protein, the vegetables provide a variety of nutrients, and the quinoa adds protein and fiber. This balanced meal supports your nutritional needs while keeping you satisfied.

Embracing a gluten-free diet might seem challenging initially. Still, with the proper knowledge and preparation, it can become second nature. Focus on naturally gluten-free foods, be vigilant about hidden sources of gluten, and ensure your meals are nutrient-dense. By doing so, you can manage celiac disease effectively and enjoy a diverse and delicious diet.

∼

NUTRITIONAL SUPPORT FOR PSORIASIS

Living with psoriasis can be a daily struggle, but the proper diet can help manage symptoms and improve skin health. Fatty fish such as salmon and sardines are rich in omega-3 fatty acids, which have been shown to reduce inflammation. These healthy fats can help alleviate the redness, itching, and scaling associated with psoriasis. Incorporating fatty fish into your diet a few times a week can make a significant difference. You can enjoy them grilled, baked, or even in a salad. Not only are they delicious, but they also provide numerous health benefits that go beyond skin health.

Colorful fruits and vegetables are another essential component of a psoriasis-friendly diet. Foods like berries, bell peppers, and leafy greens contain antioxidants that help fight inflammation and oxidative stress. Antioxidants neutralize free radicals, which can damage cells and exacerbate psoriasis symptoms. By filling your plate with a rainbow of fruits and vegetables, you can give your body the nutrients it needs to support skin health. These foods are versatile and can be included in smoothies, salads, stir-fries, or enjoyed as snacks.

While adding anti-inflammatory foods is beneficial, avoiding foods that can trigger or worsen psoriasis flare-ups is equally essential. Dairy products are one such category that can be inflammatory for some individuals. If your symptoms worsen after consuming dairy, consider reducing or eliminating it. Instead, opt for dairy alternatives like almond milk or coconut yogurt, which can provide similar textures and flavors without the inflammatory effects. Nightshade vegetables, such as tomatoes, peppers, and eggplants, can also be problematic for some people with psoriasis. These vegetables contain alkaloids that may trigger inflammation in sensitive individuals. If you suspect nightshades are affecting your symptoms, try eliminating them for a few weeks to see if your condition improves.

Supporting skin health through diet involves more than

just reducing inflammation. Certain nutrients are particularly beneficial for maintaining healthy skin. Vitamin A, found in sweet potatoes and carrots, promotes cell turnover and repair in skin health. Including these vibrant vegetables in your diet can help keep your skin looking healthy and reduce the severity of psoriasis symptoms. Zinc is another vital nutrient for skin health. It supports immune function and helps reduce inflammation. Foods like pumpkin seeds and chickpeas are excellent sources of zinc. Add pumpkin seeds to your salads or enjoy chickpeas in various dishes, from hummus to stews.

Hydration is also vital to managing psoriasis. Drinking plenty of water helps keep your skin hydrated and can reduce dryness and itching. Aim to drink at least half your body weight in ounces of water daily, and consider incorporating herbal teas into your routine. Teas like chamomile, peppermint, and green tea have anti-inflammatory properties. They can be soothing for both your skin and digestive system. Hydrating foods like cucumbers and watermelon can also support your hydration efforts. These foods have high water content and can be easily added to salads or enjoyed as refreshing snacks.

In addition to dietary changes, proper skin care is essential for managing psoriasis. Gentle, fragrance-free cleansers and moisturizers can help maintain the skin's barrier and prevent irritation. Oatmeal baths can soothe itching and reduce inflammation. Protecting your skin from the sun is essential by using sunscreen and wearing protective clothing. While a certain amount of sun exposure can benefit psoriasis, too much can lead to sunburn and worsen symptoms. By combining dietary strategies with proper skin care, you can effectively manage psoriasis and improve your overall quality of life.

This chapter explored how targeted dietary strategies can help manage various autoimmune conditions, from rheumatoid arthritis to psoriasis. You can take significant steps toward better health by making informed food choices and understanding the impact of different nutrients. Next, we'll delve into the holistic approach to managing autoimmune diseases, integrating diet with lifestyle changes to support your overall well-being. See Bonus Link for continued Autoimmunes list:

https://docs.google.com/document/d/1LRxLxICD6-H0erU0aUmgT18xWuG_w9SSKAyhaZWqkEY/edit?usp=sharing

MAKE A DIFFERENCE WITH YOUR REVIEW

Unlock the Power of Generosity

"The best way to find yourself is to lose yourself in the service of others." - Mahatma Gandhi

Helping others makes life better, don't you think? Let's make a difference together!

Would you help someone just like you—someone curious about how to live better with autoimmune disease but unsure where to begin?

My goal with *The Autoimmune Anti-Inflammatory Diet for Beginners* is to make managing autoimmune disease easier and more empowering for everyone.

But I need your help to reach more people. Most of us pick books based on reviews, and a simple review from you could make a huge difference for someone starting their wellness journey.

It costs nothing, takes just a minute, but could help...

...one more person begin a path to better health.

...one more family member support their loved one with confidence.

...one more person find hope and comfort on their wellness journey.

...one more reader discover they're not alone.

...one more life transformed.

To make a difference, just scan the QR code below or follow this link to leave a review:

Bonus recipe Link Material:

https://docs.google.com/document/d/1LRxLxICD6-H0erU0aUmgT18xWuG_w9SSKAyhaZWqkEY/edit?usp=sharing

If you love helping others, you're my kind of person. Thank you from the bottom of my heart!

T. Sherbrook

CHAPTER SIX

THE HOLISTIC APPROACH TO MANAGING AUTOIMMUNE DISEASES

When Clara first learned she had lupus, she felt a wave of anxiety wash over her. The diagnosis was daunting, not just because of the physical symptoms but also due to the emotional toll it took on her. Clara noticed that her symptoms worsened during stressful periods, such as when she had tight work deadlines or personal conflicts. Determined to find relief, she began exploring how managing stress could help her condition. This chapter delves into stress's profound impact on autoimmune diseases and offers practical strategies for managing it.

∼

THE ROLE OF STRESS MANAGEMENT

Understanding how chronic stress exacerbates autoimmune conditions is crucial. Stress is more than just feeling overwhelmed; it triggers a cascade of physiological responses that can wreak havoc on your body. When stressed, your body releases stress hormones like cortisol and adrenaline. These hormones prepare you for a "fight or flight" response, which is helpful in short bursts but harmful when prolonged. Chronic stress keeps your body heightened, leading to increased inflammation, which can worsen autoimmune symptoms. For instance, research has shown that individuals with stress-related disorders, such as PTSD, have a higher incidence of autoimmune diseases. This connection underscores the importance of addressing stress as part of your holistic health approach.

The physiological effects of stress on the immune system are significant. Chronic stress can weaken your immune response, making you more susceptible to infections and exacerbating autoimmune conditions. Stress hormones like cortisol can suppress the immune system's effectiveness by reducing the production of lymphocytes, a type of white blood cell that fights off infections. Additionally, chronic stress can increase the production of pro-inflammatory cytokines, which are proteins that promote inflammation. The heightened inflammatory state can lead to flare-ups in autoimmune conditions, making it essential to manage stress effectively to keep inflammation under control.

Effective stress management techniques can significantly improve your quality of life. One simple yet powerful technique is deep breathing. Taking slow, deep breaths activates your body's relaxation response, which helps reduce stress hormones and lower your heart rate. Progressive muscle relaxation is another effective method. This technique involves tensing and slowly relaxing different muscle groups in your body, which can help release physical tension and calm your mind. Time management strategies are also crucial. By organizing your daily tasks and setting realistic goals, you can reduce the feeling of being overwhelmed, allowing you to manage stress more effectively.

Stress management in your daily life requires consistent effort but can yield profound benefits. Setting aside time each day for relaxation is a good starting point. Whether it's a few minutes of meditation in the morning or a calming bath before bed, these small practices can make a big difference. Creating a calming bedtime routine can also help. Dim the lights, put away electronic devices, and engage in relaxing activities like reading or listening to soothing music. Finding hobbies that reduce stress, such as gardening, painting, or yoga, can provide a much-needed break from daily pressures and help you unwind.

Monitoring your stress levels is essential to understand how stress affects you and to identify patterns. Keeping a stress diary can be a helpful tool. In this diary, note moments you feel stressed and what triggered those feelings. Over time, you may notice patterns that can help you identify and address specific stressors. Recognizing physical and emotional signs of stress is also essential. Physical signs might include headaches, muscle tension, or digestive issues. In contrast, emotional signs can range from irritability to feelings of anxiety or sadness. Knowing these signs, you can take proactive steps to manage your stress before it becomes overwhelming.

Reflection Section: Stress Diary Exercise

Take a few minutes daily to jot down any stressful events or feelings you experienced. Note the time, your emotional response, and any physical symptoms. Reflect on patterns or triggers that emerge over a week. Use this insight to develop personalized strategies for managing stress, such as avoiding specific triggers or incorporating more relaxation techniques into your routine.

In sum, understanding and managing stress is critical to living well with an autoimmune condition. Incorporating effective stress management techniques into your daily life can reduce inflammation, improve your immune function, and enhance your overall well-being. *Clara's journey with lupus taught her that controlling stress was not just beneficial but essential for managing her symptoms and improving her quality of life.* Taking these steps can help you achieve similar benefits, empowering you to take control of your health.

∽

IMPORTANCE OF QUALITY SLEEP

When managing autoimmune diseases, the importance of quality sleep cannot be overstated. Sleep is a fundamental pillar of good health, critical in regulating the immune system. During sleep, your body goes through various essential stages for immune function. During these stages, your body produces and releases cytokines, a type of protein that targets infection and inflammation. Without adequate sleep, the production of these protective cytokines decreases, weakening your immune response. Weakening your immune system can make you more susceptible to infections and exacerbate autoimmune symptoms. Poor sleep can also lead to increased levels of stress hormones like cortisol, which can further elevate inflammation in the body.

Creating a sleep-friendly environment is a practical way to improve the quality of your rest. Start by keeping your bedroom cool, dark, and quiet. A room that is too warm or noisy can disrupt sleep, making reaching the deep stages necessary for restorative rest difficult. Invest in a comfortable mattress and pillows that support your body well. A good mattress can significantly affect how well you sleep and how you feel when you wake up. Consider blackout curtains to keep the room dark, and use a white noise machine if external sounds are a problem. These changes can create a sanctuary that promotes better sleep.

Healthy sleep hygiene practices are crucial for maintaining a regular sleep pattern. Establishing a consistent sleep schedule by going to bed and waking up at the same time daily can help regulate your body's internal clock. Avoid screens and caffeine at least an hour before bedtime, as the blue light from devices can interfere with the production of melatonin, a hormone that regulates sleep. Instead, relax before bed, such as reading a book, taking a warm bath, or practicing gentle yoga. These activities can signal to your body that it is time to wind down, making falling and staying asleep easier.

Dealing with sleep disorders is another crucial aspect of achieving quality sleep. Insomnia, characterized by difficulty falling or staying asleep, is a common issue that can significantly impact your quality of life. Signs of insomnia include:

- • Lying awake for long periods.
- • Waking up frequently during the night.

- - Feeling tired despite spending enough time in bed.

Sleep apnea, a condition in which breathing repeatedly stops and starts during sleep, is another disorder that can disrupt rest. Common signs of sleep apnea include loud snoring, gasping for air during sleep, and excessive daytime sleepiness. If you suspect you have a sleep disorder, it is important to consult a healthcare professional. They can provide a proper diagnosis and recommend treatments such as cognitive behavioral therapy for insomnia or continuous positive airway pressure (CPAP) therapy for sleep apnea.

Recognizing and addressing sleep disorders can significantly improve your overall health and well-being. For instance, if you frequently wake up feeling unrefreshed or your partner notices you snore loudly or gasp for air during sleep, these could be signs of sleep apnea. Consulting a healthcare professional can help you get the proper treatment, improve your sleep, and reduce the risk of complications associated with untreated sleep disorders. In the case of insomnia, techniques like cognitive behavioral therapy can help you identify and change behaviors and thoughts that negatively impact your sleep. By addressing these issues, you can improve your sleep quality and, in turn, better manage your autoimmune condition.

Quality sleep is a cornerstone of managing autoimmune diseases, as it supports immune function and helps keep inflammation in check. By creating a sleep-friendly environment, practicing good sleep hygiene, and addressing any sleep disorders, you can significantly improve the quality of your rest. These changes can lead to better overall health, reduced symptoms, and greater well-being.

INCORPORATING GENTLE EXERCISE

When diagnosed with an autoimmune condition, the thought of exercising might seem overwhelming or even daunting. However, gentle exercise can offer numerous benefits for your health. Engaging in regular, low-impact physical activities helps reduce inflammation and improve mobility. Movement can aid in maintaining joint flexibility and reducing stiffness, which is particularly beneficial for conditions like rheumatoid arthritis. Additionally, exercise stimulates the production of anti-inflammatory molecules, supporting overall immune function. Beyond physical benefits, exercise can boost your mood and energy levels. Endorphins, often called "feel-good" hormones, are released during physical activity, helping to alleviate symptoms of depression and anxiety frequently associated with chronic illness.

Several types of gentle exercises are particularly suitable for individuals with autoimmune conditions. Yoga is an excellent choice, offering both physical and mental benefits. The gentle stretching and poses in yoga help improve flexibility and joint health while promoting relaxation and reducing stress. Pilates, similar to yoga, focuses on core strength, stability, and controlled movements, which can enhance posture and balance. Swimming and water aerobics are fantastic options, too. The buoyancy of water reduces the strain on joints, making it easier to move and exercise without causing pain. Walking and light hiking are also effective, providing cardiovascular benefits and promoting overall fitness without the high impact of running or intense workouts.

Creating a sustainable exercise routine begins with setting realistic goals and starting slowly. It's essential to listen to your body and recognize your limits. Begin with short sessions, 10 to 15 minutes, and gradually increase the duration as you build strength and stamina. Incorporate exercise into your daily activities to make it more manageable. For example, take a brisk walk during your lunch break or do a few yoga stretches while watching TV. Consistency is key, so aim to move daily, even if it's just a short stroll around your neighborhood.

Listening to your body is crucial when managing an autoimmune condition. Pay attention to how you feel during and after exercise. If you experience increased pain or fatigue, it may indicate that you've overexerted yourself. Recognizing signs of overexertion, such as persistent soreness, extreme tiredness, or worsening symptoms, is essential. Balancing rest and activity is vital for maintaining your health. On days when you feel more energetic, you might engage in a longer or more vigorous session. Conversely, on days when your symptoms are more pronounced, opt for gentler activities or take a rest day. This balance helps prevent burnout and supports long-term adherence to your exercise routine.

Incorporating exercise into your routine doesn't have to be a chore. Find activities that you enjoy and that fit seamlessly into your life. For instance, if you love nature, opt for outdoor walks or hikes. If you prefer social activities, join a group class or exercise with a friend. The goal is to move regularly and make it an enjoyable part of your day. Remember, the benefits of gentle exercise go beyond physical health. It can become a time for self-care, a moment to focus on your well-being, and an opportunity to connect with your body positively.

The benefits of gentle exercise extend beyond just managing symptoms. Regular physical activity can improve your overall quality of life, making day-to-day activities more manageable and enjoyable. For example, increased flexibility and strength can help you carry groceries, climb stairs, or play with your children without pain or discomfort. Moreover, the mental health benefits of exercise, such as reduced anxiety and improved mood, can significantly enhance your emotional well-being. When you feel better mentally, you're more likely to engage in other healthy behaviors, creating a positive cycle that supports your overall health.

By incorporating gentle exercise into your routine, you can take proactive steps to manage your autoimmune condition effectively. Whether it's yoga, swimming, or a daily walk, these activities offer a range of physical and mental benefits that support your health. Listen to your body, start slow, and find activities you enjoy. With consistency and balance, you can make exercise a valuable part of your holistic approach to managing autoimmune diseases.

∼

MINDFULNESS AND MEDITATION PRACTICES

Integrating mindfulness and meditation into your routine can be transformative when dealing with the daily challenges of an autoimmune condition. Mindfulness is fully present in the moment, paying attention to your thoughts, feelings, and surroundings without judgment. Conversely, meditation involves focused attention and relaxation techniques to achieve a mentally clear and emotionally calm state. Both practices offer significant benefits, such as reducing stress and anxiety. By quieting the mind, you can lower the production of stress hormones like cortisol, which can exacerbate inflammation. Enhanced focus and emotional regulation are other advantages, helping you cope better with the unpredictability of autoimmune diseases.

Mindful breathing is one of the most straightforward mindfulness techniques to incorporate daily. Mindful breathing involves taking slow, deep breaths and focusing entirely on breathing. Pay attention to the sensation of the air entering and leaving your nostrils, the rise and fall of your chest, and the rhythm of your breath. Even a few minutes of mindful breathing can help calm your mind and reduce stress. Another effective technique is the body scan meditation. In this practice, you mentally scan your body from head to toe, paying attention to any areas of tension or discomfort. Meditation helps you become more aware of your physical state and encourages relaxation. Mindful eating is another practical approach. Instead of rushing through meals, take the time to savor each bite, noticing the flavors, textures, and aromas. Mindful eating not only aids digestion but also promotes a sense of mindfulness in everyday activities.

Guided meditation resources can be beneficial for those new in meditation. Popular apps like Headspace and Calm offer a variety of guided sessions tailored to different needs, from stress reduction to improved sleep. These apps provide easy-to-follow instructions, making meditating simple without prior experience. Online guided meditation videos are another valuable resource. Platforms such as YouTube offer various guided sessions, allowing you to select the duration and focus that best meet your needs. Whether you prefer a short five-minute session or a more extended, more immersive experience, these resources can help you build a consistent meditation practice.

Integrating mindfulness into your daily routine doesn't have to be complicated. Start with short meditation sessions, perhaps five minutes daily, and gradually increase the duration as you become pleasant. Consistency is vital, so try to meditate at the same time each day, whether in the morning to start your day calmly or in the evening to unwind before bed. Practicing mindfulness during routine activities can also be beneficial. For example, while walking, pay attention to the sensation of your feet touching the ground, the surrounding sounds, and the rhythm of your steps. When eating, focus on the taste and texture of your food, chewing slowly and enjoying each bite. These small practices can make a big difference in your overall well-being.

∼

INTERACTIVE ELEMENT: **Mindfulness Journal Prompt**

SET ASIDE a few minutes each day to write in a mindfulness journal. Note moments when you felt particularly present and engaged, whether during meditation, a walk, or a meal. Reflect on how these moments made you feel and any changes you noticed in your stress levels or mood. Use this journal to track your progress and identify areas to incorporate more mindfulness practices.

Mindfulness and meditation are powerful tools for managing stress and emotional challenges associated with an autoimmune condition. By incorporating these practices into daily life, you can reduce stress, enhance emotional regulation, and improve your overall quality of life. Taking the time to be present and mindful can provide a much-needed respite from the demands of daily life, allowing you to focus on your well-being and find a sense of peace and balance.

∼

NATURAL REMEDIES AND SUPPLEMENTS

Natural remedies can significantly manage autoimmune symptoms, offering a holistic approach to complement conventional treatments. Herbal teas are popular for many, providing both soothing effects and health benefits. Chamomile tea, for instance, is known for its calming properties, which can help ease anxiety and improve sleep quality. Peppermint tea, conversely, can aid digestion and reduce symptoms like bloating and gas, which are common in autoimmune conditions. These teas are easy to prepare and can be a comforting addition to your daily routine.

Essential oils are another natural remedy that can support your well-being. Aromatherapy uses these oils to promote physical and emotional health. For example, lavender oil is renowned for its ability to reduce stress and promote relaxation. Adding a few drops to a diffuser or a warm bath can help create a calming environment. Eucalyptus oil, known for its anti-inflammatory properties, can relieve respiratory issues or muscle pain. Simply inhaling the steam from a bowl of hot water with a few drops of eucalyptus oil can provide relief. You can incorporate essential oils into daily life through diffusers, topical applications, or bath soaks.

Evidence-based supplements can also support autoimmune health. Turmeric, a spice commonly used in cooking, contains curcumin, a compound with powerful anti-inflammatory effects. Studies have shown that curcumin can help reduce inflammation and pain in conditions like rheumatoid arthritis. A curcumin supplement can be more effective than turmeric alone, as it provides a concentrated dose. Probiotics are another valuable supplement, promoting gut health by balancing the beneficial bacteria in your digestive system. A healthy gut microbiome is crucial for immune function and can help reduce inflammation. Look for probiotic supplements that contain various strains for the best results.

Omega-3 fatty acids are essential for immune modulation and reducing inflammation. Healthy fats found in fatty fish like salmon and mackerel, as well as in flaxseeds and walnuts, omega-3s can help manage autoimmune symptoms. If getting enough omega-3s from your diet is challenging, consider taking a fish oil supplement. These supplements are widely available and can provide the necessary amounts of EPA and DHA, the active forms of omega-3s. Incorporating these supplements into your daily routine can support overall health and help manage your condition more effectively.

Before starting any new supplement, it's essential to consult your healthcare provider. Supplements can interact with medications you're taking, potentially causing adverse effects. For example, turmeric supplements can interact with blood thinners, increasing the risk of bleeding. Your healthcare provider can help determine the appropriate dosage and ensure the supplements are safe. They can also monitor your progress and adjust as needed, providing personalized care tailored to your needs.

Integrating natural remedies into your daily life can be simple and effective. Start by creating a daily supplement routine. Set a specific time each day to take your supplements, whether with breakfast or before bed. This consistency can help you remember to take them regularly and maximize their benefits. Essential oils for relaxation and stress relief can also become part of your daily routine. Diffuse calming oils like lavender in the evening to create a peaceful atmosphere, or apply diluted oils to your wrists and temples for a quick stress-relief boost during the day.

Natural remedies and supplements can offer valuable support in managing autoimmune conditions. Incorporating herbal teas, essential oils, and evidence-based supplements into your routine can enhance your overall well-being and complement your existing treatment plan. Always consult your healthcare provider before starting new supplements to ensure they are safe and appropriate. With a thoughtful approach, natural remedies can become a beneficial part of your holistic health strategy.

BUILDING A SUPPORT SYSTEM

Living with an autoimmune disease can often feel isolating, but having a solid support system can make a world of difference. Emotional support is crucial, as feeling understood and validated by others can alleviate the mental

THE AUTOIMMUNE ANTI-INFLAMMATORY DIET FOR BE...

burden of chronic illness. When you know that people around you empathize with your struggles, it can reduce feelings of loneliness and depression. Emotional support also fosters resilience, helping you cope better with the ups and downs of your condition. Beyond emotional benefits, practical assistance with daily tasks and healthcare management can provide much-needed relief. A robust support network can significantly lighten your load, whether it's help with household chores, attending medical appointments, or just having someone to talk to.

Finding support networks is an essential step in building this foundation. Local and online support groups offer a safe space to share experiences, seek advice, and find camaraderie among people who understand what you're going through. Local groups often meet regularly, providing face-to-face interaction and a sense of community. Online support groups, on the other hand, offer the convenience of connecting anytime, anywhere. Platforms like Facebook and specialized forums can connect you with like-minded individuals with similar challenges. Social media also provides opportunities to join communities focused on autoimmune diseases, where you can find resources, encouragement, and even make friends.

Another critical component is communicating effectively with loved ones about your needs and boundaries. Being open about the challenges of living with an autoimmune disease can foster understanding and empathy. Share your experiences honestly, explaining how specific symptoms affect your daily life. This transparency helps loved ones grasp the realities of your condition and respond more supportively. When you need particular types of support, don't hesitate to ask. Whether you need help with grocery shopping, want someone to accompany you to a doctor's appointment, or need a listening ear, clear communication can ensure you get the support you need. Setting boundaries is equally important. Let your loved ones know when you need rest or personal space, and remind them that these boundaries are essential for your well-being.

Professional support can also play a vital role. Working with a therapist or counselor can provide a safe space to explore your emotions, develop coping strategies, and improve your mental health. A therapist can help you navigate the emotional challenges of living with a chronic condition, offering tools to manage stress, anxiety, and depression. Consulting a nutritionist or health coach can provide personalized dietary advice tailored to your needs. These professionals can help you develop a nutrition plan that supports your health goals, considering any dietary restrictions or preferences you may have. They can also offer guidance on meal planning, grocery shopping, and cooking, making adhering to an anti-inflammatory diet easier.

Building a support system involves seeking help and creating connections with others who can offer emotional, practical, and professional support. You can build a robust network that supports your well-being by joining support networks, communicating effectively with loved ones, and seeking professional guidance. This foundation of support is not just a safety net but a critical aspect of managing your autoimmune condition effectively. It can provide the strength and resilience needed to face daily challenges and improve your quality of life.

With a robust support system in place, you can better navigate the complexities of living with an autoimmune disease. This chapter has explored how social connections, open communication, and professional support can make a significant difference. As you continue this path, remember that you don't have to do it alone. The next chapter will delve into empowering your health journey, focusing on actionable steps and practical advice to take control of your well-being.

∼

CHAPTER
SEVEN
EMPOWERING YOUR HEALTH JOURNEY

When Tom first felt the persistent joint pain, he dismissed it as a sign of aging. But as the pain intensified and fatigue set in, he realized something more serious might be at play. After multiple doctor visits and a diagnosis of an autoimmune disease, Tom felt lost. The medical jargon was overwhelming, and he wondered how to regain control of his health. This chapter is for individuals like Tom, seeking to understand their bodies better and make informed health decisions.

∽

LISTENING TO YOUR BODY

Understanding your body's signals is crucial in managing an autoimmune condition. Often, your body communicates through symptoms, which can serve as early warnings that something is amiss. Fatigue, for instance, is not just a result of a busy day; it can indicate that your body is fighting inflammation. Similarly, persistent joint pain isn't merely a nuisance but a sign that your immune system might attack your joints. Recognizing these signs early can help you take proactive steps to manage your condition better.

Digestive discomforts can also indicate how your body responds to certain foods. Bloating, gas, and irregular bowel movements can signal that your current diet includes items that do not agree with your system. Identifying these triggers is the first step in adjusting your diet to reduce inflammation and promote gut health. For instance, dairy and gluten are common culprits that can exacerbate digestive issues in individuals with autoimmune diseases. You can make more informed dietary choices by observing how your body reacts after eating certain foods.

The mind-body connection plays a vital role in managing autoimmune diseases. Stress and mental health directly influence physical symptoms. Chronic stress can elevate cortisol levels and increase inflammation, making stress management a critical component of your health strategy. Techniques like meditation and mindfulness can significantly enhance your mind-body awareness. Meditation helps calm the mind, reducing stress and its harmful effects on the body. Mindfulness involves staying present and fully engaging with the moment, which can help you become more aware of your body's needs and responses.

Adjusting your diet based on your body's feedback is another powerful way to manage your health. Start by eliminating foods that cause adverse reactions. If you notice that consuming dairy products leads to bloating and discomfort, consider removing them from your diet. Similarly, if gluten triggers joint pain or fatigue, try a gluten-free diet and observe any changes. Introducing new foods gradually allows you to monitor their effects on your symptoms. For example, add a new vegetable or fruit to your diet and see how your body responds. This method helps you identify which foods support your health and which you should avoid.

Awareness of your body's signals empowers you to make informed health decisions. Keeping a symptom journal is an effective tool for tracking changes and patterns. Document what you eat, how you feel, and any symptoms you experience. Over time, you'll notice trends that can guide your dietary and lifestyle choices. Consult healthcare professionals for tailored advice if you observe consistent reactions to specific foods or stressors. Your healthcare provider can help you interpret these patterns and develop a personalized plan to manage your condition.

Remember, you are your best advocate. Understanding and listening to your body lets you control your health. By recognizing signs of inflammation, identifying dietary triggers, and enhancing your mind-body connection, you can make proactive choices that improve your well-being. Maintaining a symptom journal and seeking professional guidance based on observations will further support your health journey. This chapter aims to empower you with the knowledge and tools to listen to your body and make informed decisions that enhance your quality of life.

∽

KEEPING A HEALTH AND FOOD DIARY

A detailed health and food diary can be a game-changer when managing an autoimmune condition. One key benefit is the ability to identify food sensitivities and intolerances. Documenting everything you eat lets you see patterns that might not have been obvious. For example, you may experience bloating, fatigue, or joint pain after eating certain foods. By tracking your food intake and symptoms, you can pinpoint foods that trigger adverse reactions and remove them from your diet.

Monitoring the impact of dietary changes on your symptoms is another significant advantage of maintaining a food diary. When you introduce new foods or eliminate potential triggers, you can observe how these changes affect your overall well-being. For instance, if you switch to a gluten-free diet and find that your joint pain diminishes, documenting this change helps confirm the positive impact of your dietary adjustments. This process not only aids in symptom management but also reinforces the benefits of making healthy choices, motivating you to stick with your new eating habits.

A comprehensive food diary should include several key elements to ensure it provides valuable insights. Start by recording your daily food intake, noting everything you eat, drink, and portion sizes. Keeping track helps you see the complete picture of your diet and identify any areas for improvement. Additionally, track your symptoms throughout the day, including any changes in mood or energy levels. This information can help you correlate specific foods with how you feel, making it easier to identify triggers. Don't forget to include physical activity and sleep patterns, as these factors can also influence your symptoms and overall health.

Using a food diary can help you stay accountable for your dietary goals. Reviewing your entries often allows you to identify patterns and areas to adjust. For example, you notice that you tend to overeat during late-night snacks. In that case, you can set a goal to have healthier options or change your meal times. Setting weekly or monthly goals based on your diary insights can keep you focused and motivated. These goals include trying new anti-inflammatory recipes, increasing your intake of specific nutrients, or reducing your consumption of processed foods.

Several tools and resources can make keeping a food diary easier and more effective. Mobile apps like MyFitnessPal and Cronometer are excellent options for tracking your food intake and nutrients. These apps often have features that allow you to scan barcodes, making it quick and easy to record what you eat. They can also provide insights into your daily caloric intake, macronutrient balance, and micronutrient levels. Printable templates are available for manual tracking if you prefer a more hands-on approach. Customize templates to fit your needs, including categories most relevant to your needs, such as specific symptoms or supplements you are taking.

If you want to take the guesswork out of figuring out which foods your body reacts to specifically, try an IGg, IGa food sensitivity test, which is available on Amazon. Make sure it tests for 96 foods or more.

Here's a simple template for your food diary to get you started. Create a table with columns for date, meal, food and portion size, symptoms, mood, physical activity, and sleep quality. Use this template daily to track your intake and observe patterns over time.

Incorporating a food diary into your daily routine can empower you to take control of your health. You can make informed decisions that support your well-being by identifying food sensitivities, monitoring dietary changes, and staying accountable. Consistency is key in using a mobile app or a printed template. Regularly reviewing your entries and setting achievable goals will help you stay on track and make meaningful progress. This practice enhances your understanding of how food impacts your body and fosters a proactive approach to managing your autoimmune condition.

∽

REAL-LIFE SUCCESS STORIES

Real-life success stories can be a powerful source of inspiration and motivation. *Consider the story of Anna, a woman diagnosed with lupus at the age of 28. Her life was filled with constant flare-ups, debilitating fatigue, and joint pain. Doctors prescribed various medications, but Anna wanted a more natural approach to complement her treatment. She started researching anti-inflammatory diets and decided to change her eating habits significantly. Anna noticed substantial improvements by eliminating processed foods and incorporating leafy greens, fatty fish, and various fruits and vegetables. Her energy levels increased, and the frequency of her flare-ups decreased. Anna's story highlights how dietary changes can make a tangible difference in managing autoimmune conditions.*

Another compelling story is that of David, who was diagnosed with rheumatoid arthritis (RA) in his early 40s. His condition made it challenging to engage in activities he once loved, such as hiking and playing with his children. David overhauled his diet, focusing on anti-inflammatory foods like turmeric, ginger, and omega-3-rich fish. He also adopted a regular exercise routine that included gentle yoga and swimming. These changes didn't come without challenges. David faced social pressures, especially during family gatherings with abundant unhealthy food choices. However, he remained committed, often sharing his anti-inflammatory dishes. Over time, David's symptoms improved, allowing him to regain a sense of normalcy.

Overcoming challenges is a common theme in these success stories. Many individuals face social pressures and family dynamics, challenging sticking to a new diet. *For instance, Sarah, who has multiple sclerosis (MS), found it challenging to maintain her diet when her family was unsupportive. She dealt with comments like, "A little bit won't hurt," and faced the temptation of her favorite comfort foods. Sarah's strategy was to educate her family about the importance of her dietary choices and involve them in meal planning and preparation. By turning meal times into a family activity, she gained their support and encouraged healthier eating habits for everyone.*

Setbacks are inevitable, but how you handle them can make all the difference. *Take the example of Michael, who has Crohn's disease. He experienced several setbacks, particularly during holidays and vacations, when sticking to his diet was challenging. Michael learned to view these setbacks as temporary and focused on getting back on track as soon as possible. He kept a positive outlook and reminded himself of the long-term benefits of his dietary changes. This mindset helped him stay motivated and committed to his health plan.*

Quotes and testimonials from those who have succeeded can be incredibly motivating. *Anna says, "Changing my diet felt overwhelming at first, but the improvements in my health were worth every effort." David shares, "It's not just about eliminating foods; it's about discovering new, delicious options that make me feel well." Sarah adds, "Involving my family made all the difference. They became my biggest supporters."*

Learning from others' experiences can provide practical tips and strategies. Many success story participants recommend starting with small, manageable changes rather than attempting an overhaul all at once. They also stress the importance of planning and preparing meals in advance to avoid last-minute, unhealthy choices. Building a community of support, whether through local groups or online forums, can offer encouragement and shared experiences that make the journey less lonely.

These stories show that while managing autoimmune diseases through diet and lifestyle changes can be challenging, it is possible and rewarding. Hearing about others' successes can inspire you to stay committed, overcome obstacles, and make choices that benefit your health.

∽

OVERCOMING INITIAL RESISTANCE

Changing your diet and lifestyle can feel daunting, and it's natural to experience resistance. One of the most common reasons for resistance is the fear of giving up favorite foods. You might love your morning coffee with cream and sugar or enjoy a slice of pizza on weekends. The thought of eliminating these comfort foods can be unsettling. Doubts about the effectiveness of dietary changes also play a significant role. After all, it can be difficult to believe that what you eat can genuinely impact your health, especially when surrounded by conflicting information and quick-fix solutions.

To overcome initial resistance, start with gradual changes rather than an all-or-nothing approach. Instead of cutting out all inflammatory foods at once, eliminate one or two at a time. For instance, if you struggle with dairy, try replacing it with plant-based alternatives for a week and observe how you feel. Gradual changes make the process more manageable and less overwhelming. Seeking support from friends, family, or support groups can also make a significant difference. Sharing your goals and challenges with others who understand or are on a similar path can provide encouragement and accountability. Support groups, whether in-person or online, offer a sense of community and shared experiences that can be incredibly motivating.

Building confidence in your ability to make and sustain changes is crucial. Celebrate small successes along the way to keep your spirits high. If you've completed a week without processed foods, acknowledge that achievement. Small victories add up and boost your confidence, making it easier to stay committed. Setting realistic and achievable goals is another effective strategy. Instead of aiming to transform your entire diet overnight, focus on one aspect at a time. For example, start by incorporating more vegetables into your meals, then gradually address other areas like reducing sugar intake. Realistic goals are more attainable and less intimidating, helping you build momentum.

Shifting your mindset can also foster a positive attitude towards dietary changes. View these changes as a form of self-care rather than deprivation. Instead of focusing on what you're giving up, think about what you're gaining—better health, increased energy, and improved well-being. Reframe your perspective to see dietary adjustments as acts of kindness towards your body. Focusing on the long-term health benefits rather than short-term sacrifices can also help. Remind yourself that the effort you put in now will pay off in reduced symptoms, fewer flare-ups, and a higher quality of life. Keeping the bigger picture in mind can make daily choices more meaningful and worthwhile.

Understanding resistance is the first step to overcoming

it. The fear of losing favorite foods, doubts about effectiveness, and the challenge of making lifestyle changes are all valid concerns. However, practical strategies and the right mindset can make the transition smoother. Gradual changes, seeking support, building confidence, and shifting your perspective are all powerful tools in your arsenal. By embracing these strategies, you can overcome initial resistance and move towards a healthier, more balanced life.

∽

STAYING MOTIVATED AND CONSISTENT

Setting clear goals is crucial in maintaining motivation and consistency on your health journey. Set SMART goals—Specific, Measurable, Achievable, Relevant, and Time-bound. **For instance**, instead of saying, *"I want to eat healthier,"* you could set a goal like, *"I will add two servings of vegetables to my daily meals for the next month."* This goal is specific and provides a clear target. Another example could be, *"I will walk for 30 minutes, five days a week, for the next three months."* This goal is measurable and time-bound, making tracking progress and staying motivated easier. By setting short-term goals, such as drinking more water throughout the day, and long-term goals, like reducing inflammation markers in blood tests over six months, you create a roadmap that guides you toward better health.

Maintaining motivation over the long term requires strategies that keep you engaged and inspired. Visual reminders of your goals can be particularly effective. You might create a **vision board** with images and words representing your health aspirations. Place it somewhere you'll see daily, like your kitchen or office. Regularly reviewing and adjusting your goals is also essential. As you achieve milestones, take the time to reflect on your progress and set new targets. Goals keep your journey dynamic and prevent stagnation. Adjusting your goals based on your experiences ensures they remain relevant and challenging, helping you stay focused and driven.

Building healthy habits is another cornerstone of consistency. Creating routines that support your dietary and lifestyle changes makes it easier to stick to them. For example, establish a Sunday meal prep routine to eat more whole foods. Spend a couple of hours chopping vegetables, cooking grains, and preparing proteins for the week ahead. Prepping sets you up for success and reduces the temptation to reach for processed convenience foods. Using habit-tracking tools can further reinforce these routines. Apps like **HabitBull** or a simple habit-tracking journal can help you monitor your progress and celebrate consistency. Seeing a streak of successful days can motivate and encourage you to keep going.

Finding motivation within a community can provide the support and encouragement you need to stay on track. Joining support groups or online communities where people share similar health goals can be incredibly empowering. These groups offer a space to share progress, discuss challenges, and receive advice. Whether it's a local meetup group or an online forum, connecting with others who understand your journey can make a significant difference. Sharing your progress and challenges with others fosters a sense of accountability. It provides a network of cheerleaders who can lift you when feeling down.

Incorporating these strategies into your daily life can help you stay motivated and consistent as you work towards better health. Setting clear, achievable goals, maintaining motivation through visual reminders, and regularly reviewing your progress are all vital steps. Building healthy habits through established routines and habit-tracking tools makes it easier to stay on course. Finally, finding motivation within a supportive community provides the encouragement and accountability needed to overcome obstacles and celebrate successes. By embracing these practices, you can create a sustainable path towards improved well-being and a healthier lifestyle.

∼

CELEBRATING SMALL WINS

Celebrating small wins is crucial for long-term success when managing an autoimmune condition. These small victories boost motivation, making you feel accomplished and capable of reaching your goals. Recognizing and celebrating progress, no matter how minor, reinforces positive behavior changes. It helps create a positive feedback loop, where the satisfaction of achieving a goal motivates you to keep going. This reinforcement is essential for maintaining consistency and staying committed to your health plan.

Identifying milestones to celebrate can be a fun and motivating exercise. Completing a week or a month of consistent dietary changes is a significant achievement. **For example, if you've successfully avoided processed foods for a week, that's worth celebrating.** Noticing improvements in symptoms or energy levels is another milestone. Perhaps you've had fewer flare-ups or felt more energetic throughout the day. These are clear indicators that your efforts are paying off, and recognizing them can keep you motivated. **"Small healthy habits, such as including**

more fruits and vegetables in your meals, deserve to be celebrated."

Creative ways to celebrate small wins can make the process enjoyable and rewarding. Treat yourself to a non-food reward, such as a new book, a wellness product, or a relaxing massage. These rewards provide a sense of accomplishment without derailing your progress. Sharing your achievements with friends or family can also be incredibly fulfilling. When you tell someone about your success, you receive positive reinforcement and encouragement, boosting your motivation. You might even inspire others to make healthier choices, creating a ripple effect of positive change.

Reflecting on your progress is a powerful way to stay motivated and practice gratitude. A gratitude journal lets you document positive changes and acknowledge your efforts. Write down what you're grateful for each day, whether feeling less pain, having more energy, or simply sticking to your diet. Reflecting on your journey helps you appreciate how far you've come and recognize the personal growth you've achieved. This practice can shift your focus from what you still need to accomplish to what you've already completed, fostering a sense of contentment and motivation to continue.

Practicing gratitude and reflection can profoundly impact your mindset and overall well-being. When you take the time to acknowledge your progress and express gratitude, you cultivate a positive outlook that makes it easier to stay committed to your goals. Reflecting on your journey helps you identify patterns and lessons learned, which can guide your future efforts. It also provides an opportunity to celebrate personal growth, recognizing that every step forward, no matter how small, is a victory worth acknowledging.

Incorporating these practices into your routine can significantly improve your ability to manage an autoimmune condition. Celebrating small wins, identifying milestones, and finding creative ways to reward yourself are all strategies that can boost your motivation and reinforce positive behavior changes. Reflecting on your progress and practicing gratitude helps you maintain a positive outlook and appreciate the journey, fostering a sense of accomplishment and motivation to keep going.

CHAPTER
EIGHT
ADVANCED TIPS AND RESOURCES

When Sophia first embraced the autoimmune anti-inflammatory diet, she was overwhelmed by the sheer volume of information. She wanted to ensure every meal supported her health goals, yet she struggled to keep her meals varied and exciting. When she discovered advanced meal-planning strategies, she felt truly empowered. These strategies transformed her approach to eating, making her diet both nutritious and enjoyable. Let's explore how you can achieve the same level of confidence and creativity in your kitchen.

∼

ADVANCED MEAL PLANNING STRATEGIES

Seasonal meal planning is a game-changer for anyone looking to enhance the quality and taste of their meals while managing costs. Focusing on seasonal produce ensures that your ingredients are at their peak freshness and nutrient density. For instance, spring brings an abundance of leafy greens like spinach and kale, rich in vitamins and antioxidants. Summer offers berries, tomatoes, and zucchini, packed with flavor and nutrients. Fall is the season for root vegetables like carrots and sweet potatoes. At the same time, winter provides citrus fruits and hearty greens like collard greens.

Beyond taste and nutrition, seasonal meal planning can also be more cost-effective. Seasonal produce is often economical because it is more abundant and does not require long-distance transportation, reducing your environmental footprint. Moreover, buying local seasonal produce supports your community's farmers and reduces the need for pesticides and preservatives. This approach benefits your health and promotes sustainability and community well-being.

Balancing macro and micronutrients in your meal planning is crucial for maintaining energy levels and overall health. Macros—proteins, fats, and carbohydrates—are the building blocks of your diet. Ensuring you have adequate protein helps with muscle repair and immune function. Healthy fats like those found in avocados and olive oil can support brain health and reduce inflammation. Complex carbohydrates, like whole grains and vegetables, provide sustained energy and essential fiber.

Micronutrients, including vitamins, minerals, and antioxidants, are equally essential. Vitamin C, found in citrus fruits, boosts your immune system, while vitamin D, which you can get from fortified foods or sunlight, is crucial for bone health. Iron in leafy greens and legumes supports oxygen transport in the blood. A balanced meal might include a quinoa salad with mixed greens, cherry tomatoes, chickpeas, and a lemon-tahini dressing, covering a wide range of nutrients in one dish.

Storing and repurposing leftovers creatively can save you time and reduce food waste. For example, roast various vegetables and use them throughout the week in different ways—perhaps in a quinoa bowl one day, a wrap the next, and a side dish for dinner. You can also make a big pot of soup or stew and freeze individual portions for future meals. This approach keeps your diet varied and interesting while ensuring you always have something healthy on hand.

To prevent dietary boredom, incorporate variety into your meal plans by rotating different cuisines and flavors. Experiment with new ingredients and recipes to keep things exciting. For instance, you might try a Mediterranean-inspired meal one night with grilled fish, olives, and a fresh salad and an Asian-inspired dish another night with stir-fried vegetables, tofu, and a sesame-ginger sauce. Theme nights, like **"Mediterranean Monday"** or **"Taco Tuesday,"** can add a fun and structured way to introduce variety to your weekly meals.

Using a theme can also make meal planning enjoyable and less of a chore. For example, on **"Mediterranean Monday,"** you could prepare dishes like hummus, tabbouleh, and grilled chicken kebabs. On **"Taco Tuesday,"** you might make tacos with black beans, avocado, and salsa. These themes can inspire you to explore new recipes and ingredients, keeping your meals delicious and nutritionally balanced.

By adopting these advanced meal planning strategies, you can create a diet that supports your health goals and is diverse and enjoyable. Embrace the benefits of seasonal produce, balance your macro and micronutrients, use batch cooking, and incorporate variety to keep your meals exciting. These practices will help you maintain a sustainable and satisfying anti-inflammatory diet.

∼

SOURCING QUALITY INGREDIENTS

Sourcing local and organic ingredients can significantly enhance the quality of your meals and support your health goals. By choosing local and organic produce, you reduce your exposure to pesticides and chemicals, often used heavily in conventional farming. These chemicals can exacerbate inflammation and other symptoms of autoimmune diseases. Local and organic foods are typically fresher because they don't have to travel long distances to reach your table. Local farm foods mean they retain more of their nutrients and natural flavors. Additionally, buying locally supports farmers in your community, promotes sustainable agriculture, and strengthens the local economy. You also contribute to environmental sustainability by reducing the carbon footprint of transporting food over long distances.

Farmers' markets and Community Supported Agriculture (CSA) programs are excellent resources for sourcing fresh, local produce. Farmers' markets are usually held weekly and bring together local farmers and producers in one location, offering various seasonal fruits, vegetables, meats, and dairy products. Check local listings or community bulletin boards to find a nearby farmers' market. Visiting a farmers' market can be a delightful experience, allowing you to interact directly with farmers, ask questions about their growing practices, and receive tips on preparing seasonal produce. CSAs offer a different model where you subscribe to receive a share of the farm's produce regularly, usually weekly or bi-weekly. CSAs ensure a steady supply of fresh, seasonal produce and support farmers by providing a reliable income stream. Joining a CSA can introduce you to new vegetables and fruits you might not have tried before, expanding your culinary horizons.

For those who prefer the convenience of online shopping, several reputable websites specialize in organic and non-GMO products. Websites like **Thrive Market** offer organic groceries, including pantry staples, snacks, and wellness products. Specialty online stores focus on unique herbs, spices, and other high-quality ingredients that might be difficult to find locally. These sites often provide detailed information about the sourcing and quality of their products, helping you make informed choices. When shopping online, look for certifications that indicate high-quality standards, such as USDA Organic, Non-GMO Project Verified, and Fair Trade Certified. These certifications ensure that the products meet specific criteria for organic farming, non-GMO ingredients, and ethical sourcing practices.

Reading labels and understanding certifications is crucial for making informed choices about the ingredients you purchase. Organic certification means that it is produced without synthetic pesticides, fertilizers, or genetically modified organisms (GMOs). The Non-GMO Project Verified label indicates that the product has been tested and confirmed to be free of GMOs. Fair Trade Certified products ensure that the farmers and workers involved in the production process are treated fairly and receive fair wages. When selecting oils and grains, choose high-quality options like extra virgin olive oil or cold-pressed avocado oil, which retain more nutrients and have anti-inflammatory properties. Opt for whole grains like quinoa, farro, and brown rice, which are less processed and provide more fiber and nutrients than refined grains. Avoid misleading labels and marketing terms that can make unhealthy products seem healthy. Terms like **"natural"** or **"made with whole grains"** can be deceptive, so always check the ingredient list and nutritional information.

By understanding the benefits of sourcing local and organic ingredients, utilizing farmers' markets and CSAs, exploring reputable online resources, and reading labels carefully, you can ensure that the food you bring into your home supports your health and well-being. Making informed choices about the quality of your ingredients is a decisive step towards managing autoimmune symptoms and embracing a nourishing, anti-inflammatory diet.

∾

EXPLORING ANTI-INFLAMMATORY SPICES AND HERBS

Using anti-inflammatory spices and herbs can greatly enhance your meals, providing flavor and health benefits. **Turmeric**, for example, is a powerhouse spice known for its curcumin content. Curcumin is a potent anti-inflammatory compound that can help reduce joint pain and stiffness, particularly in conditions like arthritis. Combine it with black pepper to make the most of turmeric, which enhances curcumin absorption. You can add turmeric to soups, stews, and smoothies for a vibrant color and health boost.

Ginger is another versatile spice with a range of benefits. It is known for its digestive properties, which can alleviate nausea and improve overall gut health. It's also effective in reducing inflammatory markers in the body. It would help if you used fresh ginger should be grated into stir-fries, added to teas, or blended into smoothies. Dried ginger powder is a convenient option for baking or seasoning dishes. Combining ginger with other spices like cinnamon and turmeric can create a synergistic effect, amplifying their benefits.

Cinnamon is well-regarded for its ability to regulate blood sugar levels and its high antioxidant content. It can help reduce inflammation by lowering the body's C-reactive protein (CRP) levels. Cinnamon is incredibly versatile and can be sprinkled on oatmeal, stirred into coffee, or used in baking. Ceylon cinnamon, often called "true cinnamon," is the best variety for health benefits and is safer for long-term use than the more common Cassia cinnamon.

"Storing spices in an airtight container is important to use them effectively. *"Please keep them in airtight containers away from light, heat, and moisture.'* Airtight containers help preserve their potency and flavor. Incorporating these spices into your daily cooking routine can be simple and enjoyable. For example, you can make a golden milk latte by mixing turmeric, ginger, and cinnamon with warm almond milk and a touch of honey. This soothing drink is not only delicious but also packed with anti-inflammatory properties.

Herbal teas and infusions are another excellent way to incorporate anti-inflammatory herbs into your diet. **Chamomile** tea is well-known for its calming effects and ability to reduce inflammation. It can help you relax after a long day and may improve sleep quality. To prepare chamomile tea, steep dried chamomile flowers in hot water for about five minutes, then strain and enjoy. Adding a slice of lemon or a teaspoon of honey can enhance the flavor.

Peppermint tea is another beneficial option, particularly for digestive health. It can help soothe an upset stomach and reduce irritable bowel syndrome (IBS) symptoms. To make peppermint tea, use fresh or dried peppermint leaves and steep them in hot water for five to ten minutes. You can drink it hot or chilled, depending on your preference. Combining different herbs to create custom blends can also be a fun and effective way to enjoy their benefits. For instance, a mix of chamomile, peppermint, and ginger can provide a comprehensive anti-inflammatory boost.

Growing herbs and spices at home can be a rewarding experience. Indoor herb gardens and container gardening are great options for those with limited space. **Basil, rosemary, and thyme** are excellent choices for beginners. Basil thrives in warm, sunny spots and needs regular watering. Rosemary prefers well-drained soil and can be grown indoors on a sunny windowsill. Thyme is hardy and doesn't require much maintenance, making it perfect for container gardening.

When planting herbs, use high-quality potting soil and ensure your containers have good drainage. Regularly trim your herbs to encourage growth and prevent them from becoming leggy. Harvesting is simple: snip off the leaves or stems as needed, using them fresh or drying them for later use. Store herbs in airtight containers and use them throughout the year. Growing your herbs ensures you have a fresh supply at your fingertips, free from pesticides and other chemicals.

By exploring and incorporating these anti-inflammatory spices and herbs into your diet, you enhance the flavor of your meals and support your overall health. These natural remedies offer a simple and effective way to manage inflammation and improve well-being.

∽

FUNCTIONAL FOODS AND THEIR BENEFITS

Functional foods are more than just sustenance; they provide health benefits beyond essential nutrition. These foods can benefit an anti-inflammatory diet, as they often contain compounds that help reduce inflammation, support immune function, and improve overall well-being. Examples of functional foods include **kefir, kimchi**, and **chia seeds**. These foods nourish your body and improve health outcomes by addressing specific dietary needs.

Probiotic-rich foods are vital for maintaining gut health, which is crucial for managing inflammation and autoimmune conditions. Yogurt and kefir, for instance, are excellent sources of beneficial bacteria that aid digestion and enhance immune function. Kefir, a fermented milk drink, is particularly potent, offering a broader range of probiotic strains than yogurt. Fermented vegetables like sauerkraut and kimchi are also valuable additions to your diet. These foods are packed with probiotics that help balance your gut microbiome, reducing symptoms like bloating and discomfort. Making your fermented foods can be a fun and rewarding project. For instance, homemade sauerkraut requires just cabbage, salt, and time. Shred the cabbage, massage it with salt, and let it ferment in a jar for a few weeks. This simple process yields a nutrient-dense food that supports gut health.

Superfoods are another functional food category that is

particularly beneficial for reducing inflammation. **Blueberries**, for example, are high in antioxidants, which help neutralize free radicals and reduce oxidative stress. Superfoods make a great addition to smoothies, oatmeal, or even salads. **Walnuts** are another excellent choice, rich in omega-3 fatty acids with potent anti-inflammatory properties. These nuts can be added to cereals, mixed into yogurt, or eaten as a snack. Incorporating superfoods into your daily meals doesn't have to be complicated. A simple smoothie recipe might include:

- • A handful of blueberries.
- • A tablespoon of chia seeds.
- • A cup of kefir.
- • A drizzle of honey.

This nutrient-packed drink tastes great and provides a range of health benefits.

Incorporating **functional foods** into your daily meals can be straightforward, with a few practical tips. Adding **chia seeds** to your smoothies and oatmeal is a simple way to boost your omega-3s, fiber, and antioxidant intake. Chia seeds are incredibly versatile and can even be used to make chia pudding by soaking them in almond milk overnight. Kefir can easily replace yogurt or milk in your diet, providing a more diverse range of probiotics. Mix kefir into your morning smoothie, pour it over granola, or use it as a base for salad dressings. Including fermented foods as side dishes is another effective strategy. A spoonful of sauerkraut or kimchi can add a tangy kick to your meals while delivering gut-friendly probiotics. These small changes can significantly affect your overall health and well-being.

Functional foods offer a powerful way to enhance your

diet and support your health goals. You can effectively manage inflammation and improve your overall well-being by incorporating probiotic-rich foods, superfoods, and other functional ingredients into your daily meals. This approach supports your health and adds variety and flavor to your diet, making it easier to stick to your nutritional goals.

~

SCIENTIFIC STUDIES SUPPORTING THE DIET

Scientific studies provide the backbone for understanding how the autoimmune anti-inflammatory diet can improve health. Numerous studies have highlighted the role of **omega-3 fatty acids** in reducing inflammation. Research has shown that omega-3s in fatty fish like salmon can lower inflammatory markers such as C-reactive protein (**CRP**) and interleukin-6 (**IL-6**), which are often elevated in autoimmune conditions. Moreover, omega-3s can help modulate the immune system, reducing the severity of autoimmune responses. Omega-3s are a valuable addition to an anti-inflammatory diet, supported by **strong scientific evidence**.

Antioxidants also play a crucial role in reducing oxidative stress, which can exacerbate inflammation. Studies have demonstrated that antioxidants like **vitamins C** and **E** can neutralize free radicals. These molecules cause cellular damage and inflammation. For instance, a survey of the Mediterranean diet, rich in antioxidant-laden fruits and vegetables, found that it significantly reduced inflammatory markers in participants. The Mediterranean diet highlights the importance of antioxidants in managing inflammation. Still, it increases the value of a diet rich in plant-based foods.

Long-term studies on dietary patterns and autoimmune disease progression offer valuable insights. These studies often follow large groups of people over many years, examining how their diets impact the development and progression of autoimmune diseases. For example, research has shown that diets high in processed foods and refined sugars are associated with increased inflammation and a higher risk of autoimmune conditions. Conversely, diets rich in whole foods, healthy fats, and lean proteins are linked to reduced inflammation and better health outcomes. These findings provide a robust foundation for adopting an anti-inflammatory diet to manage autoimmune diseases.

Understanding research methodologies helps you critically evaluate studies and apply their findings to your life. Observational studies and clinical trials are two common types of research. Observational studies look at associations between diet and health outcomes in large populations. These studies can identify trends but can't prove cause and effect. Clinical trials, on the other hand, involve controlled experiments where participants are randomly assigned to different diet groups. These trials can demonstrate causal relationships but are often more complex and expensive. These studies' sample sizes and control groups are crucial for ensuring reliable results. A larger sample size increases the study's power. At the same time, control groups help isolate the effect of the diet from other variables. Interpreting statistical significance is also crucial—results must be statistically significant to be considered reliable, meaning the findings are unlikely to be due to chance.

Landmark research has significantly shaped our understanding of diet and inflammation. The Mediterranean diet is one of the most studied for its anti-inflammatory effects. It emphasizes whole grains, fruits, vegetables, nuts, and olive oil and includes moderate fish and poultry. Studies have shown that this diet can reduce inflammatory markers and lower the risk of chronic diseases. Another area of interest is the gut microbiota's role in autoimmune diseases. Research indicates that a healthy gut microbiome, supported by a fiber-rich diet and fermented foods, can modulate the immune system and reduce inflammation. Specific studies on dietary interventions for rheumatoid arthritis and lupus have demonstrated that anti-inflammatory diets can alleviate symptoms and improve quality of life.

Practical applications of research findings can transform your approach to meal planning and food choices. For instance, incorporating omega-3-rich foods like salmon and flaxseeds into your diet can help manage inflammation. Using research-backed supplements, such as fish oil or curcumin, can provide additional support. Staying updated with new research through reputable sources, such as scientific journals and health organizations, ensures you benefit from the latest findings. This proactive approach helps you make informed decisions, tailoring your diet to support your health and well-being.

RESOURCES FOR FURTHER LEARNING

Books and publications can be invaluable resources for navigating the autoimmune anti-inflammatory diet. Titles by experts in nutrition and autoimmune health provide in-depth knowledge and practical advice. For example, "The Anti-Inflammatory Diet and Action Plans" by Dorothy Calimeris offers comprehensive guides to managing inflammation through diet. Dr. Terry Wahls' "The Wahls Protocol" is another excellent resource detailing how specific dietary changes can alleviate autoimmune symptoms. These books often include meal plans, recipes, and scientific explanations that make complex concepts accessible and actionable. Moreover, cookbooks focused on anti-inflammatory recipes, such as "Anti-Inflammatory Eating Made Easy" by Michelle Babb, offer a variety of delicious and nutritious meal ideas. These cookbooks can help you diversify your diet while ensuring you get the nutrients you need to manage inflammation effectively.

Online courses and webinars are another excellent way to deepen your understanding of the autoimmune anti-inflammatory diet. Many institutions and health professionals offer courses on nutrition and dietetics, focusing specifically on anti-inflammatory diets. These courses range from short webinars to in-depth programs, allowing you to choose the level of detail that suits your needs. For example, websites like Coursera and Udemy feature courses on nutrition that can enhance your understanding and application of anti-inflammatory dietary principles. Webinars by healthcare professionals and researchers often cover the latest diet and autoimmune health findings, offering a convenient way to stay informed. These webinars can provide up-to-date information and practical tips to apply to your daily routine immediately.

Support groups and online communities offer ongoing support and information sharing, which can be incredibly beneficial. Online forums and social media groups provide platforms to connect with others on similar health journeys. These communities can offer practical tips, recipe ideas, and emotional support. For instance, joining a Facebook group focused on autoimmune health can give you a wealth of shared experiences and advice. Local meetups and workshops can also provide valuable opportunities for learning and connection. These gatherings allow you to meet like-minded individuals in your community, share your experiences, and learn from others who have successfully managed their conditions. Being part of a supportive community can make the process of adopting and maintaining an anti-inflammatory diet more manageable and enjoyable.

Seeking professional guidance is another essential step in managing your autoimmune condition effectively. Consulting with a registered dietitian or nutritionist can provide personalized advice tailored to your needs and health conditions. These professionals can help you develop a meal plan that aligns with your health goals, ensuring you get the necessary nutrients while managing inflammation. Working with a healthcare team, including specialists in autoimmune diseases, can offer comprehensive support, addressing all aspects of your health. Finding specialists who understand the complex nature of autoimmune conditions can make a significant difference in your treatment and management strategies. These professionals can provide the latest research-backed information and help you implement effective dietary and lifestyle changes.

Utilizing these resources can deepen your understanding of the autoimmune anti-inflammatory diet and help you gain the tools to manage your condition effectively. Whether through books, online courses, support groups, or professional guidance, these resources provide valuable insights that can help you on your path to better health. This comprehensive approach ensures that you are well-equipped to make informed decisions about your diet and lifestyle, ultimately helping you achieve improved well-being.

∼

CONCLUSION

You have taken a significant step towards better health and well-being by exploring "The Autoimmune Anti-Inflammatory Diet for Beginners." This journey is about guiding and empowering you to manage autoimmune diseases through an anti-inflammatory diet and holistic lifestyle changes. Let's revisit this book's core principles and insights to reinforce how these strategies can transform your life.

Understanding autoimmunity and inflammation is the foundation of managing autoimmune conditions. Autoimmunity occurs when your immune system mistakenly attacks your body, leading to chronic inflammation. This book has explained how inflammation, while a natural response to injury or infection, can become harmful when it persists over time. Chronic inflammation is a critical factor in autoimmune diseases, contributing to various symptoms and complications.

The autoimmune anti-inflammatory diet is central to managing these conditions. Following this diet, you incorporate anti-inflammatory foods like leafy greens, fatty fish,

CONCLUSION

and healing herbs. These foods help reduce inflammation, support immune function, and promote well-being. Equally important is understanding which foods to avoid, such as refined sugars, trans fats, and processed meats, which can trigger inflammation and worsen symptoms.

Meal planning and preparation are crucial for maintaining this diet. Practical advice on meal planning, budget-friendly shopping, and batch cooking has been provided to help you stay consistent. Managing cravings and finding healthy substitutions are vital strategies to keep you on track.

Holistic health strategies complement the diet. Stress management, quality sleep, gentle exercise, and mindfulness practices are all critical for overall health and well-being. These strategies help reduce stress-related flare-ups and support the body's natural healing processes.

Specialized dietary strategies are tailored to specific autoimmune diseases. Whether you're dealing with rheumatoid arthritis, lupus, or Hashimoto's thyroiditis, this book provides targeted nutritional recommendations to help you manage your symptoms effectively.

Inspirational success stories from individuals who have successfully managed their autoimmune diseases through diet and lifestyle changes highlight the real-life impact of these strategies. These stories are a powerful reminder that you are not alone on this journey and that positive change is possible.

Overcoming challenges is a crucial part of this journey. This book addresses common obstacles, from social pressures to initial resistance, and provides practical strategies for overcoming them. Emphasizing the importance of mindset shifts and gradual changes can help you stay motivated and committed.

CONCLUSION

Finally, advanced tips and resources have been offered to support you long-term. From seasonal meal planning, sourcing quality ingredients, exploring anti-inflammatory spices, and understanding scientific studies, these tools and strategies will help you maintain the autoimmune anti-inflammatory diet.

As you move forward, take immediate steps towards adopting the anti-inflammatory diet and lifestyle. Start by making small, manageable changes and gradually build on them. Remember, every positive change brings you closer to improved health and quality of life.

Empowering yourself with knowledge and taking control of your health can be a transformative experience. Stay committed to this journey, and don't be afraid to seek support from your community, whether it's through local groups, online forums, or professional guidance. You have the power to make a difference in your life.

In conclusion, the autoimmune anti-inflammatory diet and holistic lifestyle changes offer a comprehensive approach to managing autoimmune diseases. Following the guidance in this book can reduce inflammation, support your immune function, and improve your overall well-being. Keep listening to your body, stay informed, and embrace a healthier, inflammation-free life. Remember, you are not alone, and every step you take towards better health is worth celebrating.

Thank you for allowing me to be a part of your health journey. I am passionate about helping beginners like you overcome the challenges of managing autoimmune diseases. Together, we have explored the powerful connection between diet and disease. I hope this book has given you the clarity, depth, and practical guidance you need to succeed. Stay empowered, stay informed, and most impor-

CONCLUSION

tantly, stay committed to your health. Your journey to a better, healthier you starts now.

REFERANCES

- *List of autoimmune diseases, with symptoms and treatments* https://www.medicalnewstoday.com/articles/list-of-autoimmune-diseases
- *Regulation of Inflammation in Autoimmune Disease - PMC* https://www.ncbi.nlm.nih.gov/pmc/articles/PMC6421792/
- *The Multiple Pathways to Autoimmunity - PMC* https://www.ncbi.nlm.nih.gov/pmc/articles/PMC5791156/
- *Chronic inflammation: Why it's harmful, and how to prevent it* https://www.novanthealth.org/healthy-headlines/chronic-inflammation-why-its-harmful-and-how-to-prevent-it
- *Foods that fight inflammation* https://www.health.harvard.edu/staying-healthy/foods-that-fight-inflammation
- *Low-Grade Inflammation and Ultra-Processed Foods ...*https://www.ncbi.nlm.nih.gov/pmc/articles/PMC10058108/
- *30-Day Anti-Inflammatory Meal Plan, Created by a*

REFERENCES

Dietitian https://www.eatingwell.com/article/7866186/30-day-anti-inflammatory-meal-plan/

- *Managing autoimmune conditions with herbal medicine* https://www.endeavour.edu.au/about-us/blog/managing-autoimmune-conditions-with-herbal-medicine/
- *The 6 Best Budget-Friendly Anti-Inflammatory Foods, …* https://www.eatingwell.com/article/8024844/best-budget-friendly-anti-inflammatory-foods/
- *Ultimate List Of Meal Prep Tools* https://fitmencook.com/blog/meal-prep-tools/
- *12 Effective Ways to Manage Food Cravings* https://www.healthline.com/nutrition/how-to-stop-food-cravings
- *Eating Out? How to Stick to Your Anti-Inflammatory Diet at …* https://www.rupahealth.com/post/eating-out-how-to-stick-to-your-anti-inflammatory-diet-at-restaurants#:~:text=Choose%20dishes%20on%20the%20menu,a%20salad%20or%20steamed%20vegetables.
- *24 Anti-Inflammatory Breakfasts with 5 Ingredients or Less* https://www.eatingwell.com/anti-inflammatory-breakfast-recipes-with-5-ingredients-or-less-8638460
- *20 Anti-Inflammatory Lunches You Can Make in 10 Minutes* https://www.eatingwell.com/gallery/7967197/anti-inflammatory-lunches-in-10-minutes/
- *38 Anti-Inflammatory Dinners You Can Make in 30 Minutes* https://www.eatingwell.com/gallery/7946056/anti-inflammatory-dinner-recipes-in-30-minutes/
- *7 Best Anti-Inflammatory Ingredients for Smoothies* https://www.realsimple.com/food-recipes/recipe-collections-favorites/popular-ingredients/anti-inflammatory-smoothie-ingredients
- *Best Foods for Rheumatoid Arthritis* https://www.arthritis.org/health-wellness/treatment/treatment-plan/tracking-your-health/foods-that-can-help-ra-symptoms

REFERENCES

- *Hashimoto Diet: Overview, Foods, Supplements, and Tips* https://www.healthline.com/nutrition/hashimoto-diet
- *What Foods & Drinks to Avoid if You Have Lupus* https://wvrheumatology.com/lupus-foods-drinks-to-avoid/
- *Eating, Diet, & Nutrition for Celiac Disease - NIDDK* https://www.niddk.nih.gov/health-information/digestive-diseases/celiac-disease/eating-diet-nutrition#:~:text=nutrients%20you%20need.-,Gluten%2Dfree%20-foods,beans%20are%20safe%20to%20eat.
- *Autoimmune disease and stress: Is there a link?* https://www.health.harvard.edu/blog/autoimmune-disease-and-stress-is-there-a-link-2018071114230
- *Role of sleep deprivation in immune-related disease risk ...* https://www.nature.com/articles/s42003-021-02825-4
- *Exercise Energizes Patients With Autoimmune Disease* https://irp.nih.gov/blog/post/2023/02/exercise-energizes-patients-with-autoimmune-disease
- *Mindfulness and Physical Disease: A Concise Review - PMC* https://www.ncbi.nlm.nih.gov/pmc/articles/PMC6597336/
- *Understanding the Psychoemotional Roots of Immune ...* https://www.ifm.org/news-insights/understanding-psychoemotional-roots-immune-disease/
- *The Benefits of Food Journaling* https://nutrition.org/the-benefits-of-food-journaling/
- *Health Topics: Autoimmune Disease & Diet* https://www.forksoverknives.com/health-topics/autoimmune-diseases-and-diet/
- *5 barriers to diet change and how to overcome them* https://www.mdanderson.org/publications/focused-on-health/5-barriers-to-diet-change-and-how-to-overcome-them.h28-1593780.html

REFERANCES

- *Discover the Benefits of Seasonal Meal Planning* https://www.fvwoman.com/2023/08/seasonal-meal-planning-2/
- *9 Herbs and Spices That Fight Inflammation* https://www.healthline.com/nutrition/anti-inflammatory-herbs
- *Community Supported Agriculture (CSA) Directory* https://www.ams.usda.gov/local-food-directories/csas
- *Anti-Inflammatory Diets - StatPearls* https://www.ncbi.nlm.nih.gov/books/NBK597377/

KEEPING THE JOURNEY GOING

Now that you've got everything you need to start feeling better and managing autoimmune disease, it's time to share your knowledge with others who might need the same help.

By leaving your honest opinion of *The Autoimmune Anti-Inflammatory Diet for Beginners* on Amazon, you'll be guiding other readers to find the information they need to start their wellness journey, too.

Thank you for helping spread the knowledge! When we share our experiences, we keep the path to wellness alive—and you're helping me make that happen.

KEEPING THE JOURNEY GOING

Scan to go to the book on Amazon.

Bonus Link: https://docs.google.com/document/d/1LRxLxICD6-H0erU0aUmgT18xWuG_w9SSKAyhaZWqkEY/edit?usp=sharing

Printed in Dunstable, United Kingdom